THE OWNER'S GUIDE TO THE TEENAGE BRAIN

Derek Pugh

Cover and Interior Design: Raven Tree Design

National Library of Australia Cataloguing-in-Publication entry :

Creator: Pugh, Derek, author.

Title: The owner's guide to the teenage brain / Derek Pugh ; Khan Wilson (illustrator)

Edition: 2nd edition.

ISBN: 9780992355883 (paperback)

Notes: Includes bibliographical references and index.

Subjects: Adolescent psychology.

Teenagers--Physiology.

Identity (Psychology) in adolescence.

Other Creators/Contributors:

Wilson, Khan, illustrator.

Also by Derek Pugh

Tambora : Travels to Sumbawa and the mountain that changed the world, 2014

Turn Left at the Devil Tree, 2013

Tammy Damulkurra, 1995 (2nd edition 2013)

Contact: *derekpugh1@gmail.com*

Website: *www.derekpugh.com.au*

To Harry and Roy.
And your teenage years!

Contents

Introduction

A common saying used to run something like: *Take away everything, except the teacher, and schools are the same as they were a hundred years ago*. It meant, I think, that teachers still do the same job and that students are the same now as they always were. But it is now patently *not* true. With modern technology, expectations, behaviour, and world events impinging on school life, school is not what it was a hundred years ago. Everything has changed, and much of it has been driven by an increasing understanding of how we learn, and how to use technology to help us learn. We walk around with encyclopaedias on our phones and we can be in 24 hour electro-social contact with hundreds of people. We are thus more connected to all knowledge (and mis-knowledge) and more people, than ever before. One of the new things we need to teach is how to access and use that knowledge and to manage those contacts.

Neuroscience is still a developing field, with new knowledge about the most complex organ in our bodies being brought to light every day. Since the first edition of this book in 2011, our understanding of the brain and how it functions has grown. I am pleased to see that schools are now listening and changes have been made in the classroom, the canteen and the school yard, that are 'brain compatible' and are having positive effects on the learning of students. Simple things, like water bottles within reach, and school breakfast programs, are now common. And teachers are being taught how to differentiate their teaching to reach all students, not just the middle range.

Knowledge is power. If you are a teenager, have one in the family, or teach some, then understanding what you, or they, are going through will give you confidence and perhaps, relief in understanding what is normal.

This book does not give you permission to act badly, be irrational, or fight with your parents (as my nephew claimed after he read the first edition). Rather it will help you understand why sometimes you can't help yourself, and understand some of the strange urges you have that can be just plain weird and upsetting, or the risks that you're willing to take that you would never have dreamed taking of a few years ago.

This book is for you if you have a brain. Your brain contains more than a hundred billion cells, called neurons, which make you a thinking being. Humans are the only species, we know of, who realise that it is our brains that let us understand how we function. What an advantage that is.

In your teenage years you start a long process of 'brain rewiring' and pruning. Your brain will never have as many neurons as it once did. You may be losing up to 30,000 brain cells *per second* during this process, as those neurons you're not using are being recycled, and those you are using are strengthened. This can have weird and wonderful effects on your behaviour and the way you think. It is normal, try to enjoy it. It won't last for ever.

This book is written for you so you'll understand what's happening as your brain changes in your teenage years, and how to get the most out of it. It's hard to go it alone, the more people who understand the brain the easier it is to set yourself up to prepare and use it well, so talk to your friends, teachers, parents or brothers and sisters (if they have been through what you're going through right now, just recently, they may have insights to share).

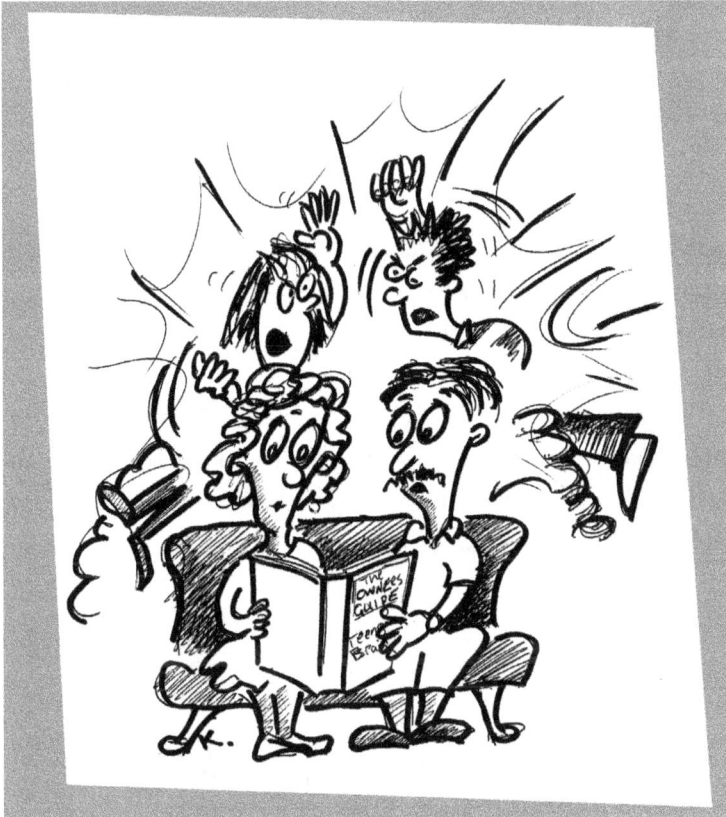

And of course, when Mum and Dad read this book they'll understand you better.

The chapters are set out in a way that takes you from the very small to the big parts of your brain and how they work, then through the 'secrets' you can adapt to suit your lifestyle and use to improve the efficiency of your brain. Using these methods you'll be able to get the best grades you can at school, develop healthy concepts and attitudes about life and understand some of the changes you've been going through like mood swings and why you're making those crazy decisions.

At the end of each chapter there are messages for both your teachers and your parents. They also need to know what you know and sometimes more, so share this book with them.

You'll meet people who are having problems with their brains. It is in all our interests that we each have some tolerance and understanding of them, what we can do to avoid some of the problems, and how to help people who have them.

Treating your brain well now is an investment that will pay dividends for the rest of your life. This book will give you the knowledge about how to do this and it will help you to make decisions that may affect you profoundly. The choices are yours to make.

Good luck.

A MESSAGE TO YOUR TEACHERS

Why should teachers know about the brain?

Knowing how the brain works can guide best teaching practices. Learners knowing how their brains work can guide choices and goals within their learning. This is powerful knowledge that can be behaviour altering, and build motivation and confidence. Teaching with the knowledge of how your students learn best and what their (and your) strengths and weaknesses are is a starting point for maximizing the return on your efforts in teaching.

Here's what some of the other writers in the field say:

Patricia Wolfe says that research adds a partial understanding of why certain procedures or strategies work – we can therefore articulate and explain the rationale for what teachers do. The brain becomes the focus of the daily work of teachers and it is no longer a 'black box'. Research can now explain a little about how it works and the better we understand it the better we can teach it. A functional understanding of the brain allows us to critically analyze the 'neuroscientific' information that arrives daily – some information is good, but some is just 'sound bytes' that invite misinterpretation or 'pseudo-science'.

Sheryl Feinstein wrote 'although you can't change teenage behaviour you *can* adapt your teaching style to effectively reach adolescents'.

David Sousa reasons that as teachers try to change human brains every day, the more they know about how it learns, the more successful they will be.

John Joseph says that young people 'will live through some of the most remarkable discoveries ever made. And, maybe not all will be to the benefit of human kind. Kids will need to be critical reviewers of research findings and apply their judgments with diligence and wisdom'.

And from Eric Jensen: 'Failing children and failing schools are an indication of a faulty system, not a faulty brain, and schools have taken enough of a beating! When students are provided with a learning environment that is optimal for learning, graduation rates increase, learning difficulties and discipline problems decrease, a love of learning flourishes… and learning organizations thrive'.

A MESSAGE TO YOUR PARENTS

Why should parents know about their teenager's brain?

Teenagers are going through massive changes. I like the analogy of teenagers being like computers – every time you go to the shop computers are more powerful, faster, with more accessories than the one you bought last month. It's hard to keep up with the changes. It's like this with our kids – every time you see your son or daughter they have progressed a little.

Knowing a little about what is going on and what to expect will help you to keep in touch with your teen and understand what he or she is going through. It's a fantastic time, but it's confusing. It's also a period of loss – your teen is no longer a child, and some parents can find it hard to 'let go' a little as their teens bid for more and more independence, and at the same time, still need guidance and support.

Section 1.
Brain Structure and Function

Chapter 1

What's it Made of?

IN THIS CHAPTER YOU WILL LEARN

* About brain cells
* Ten parts of the brain you can easily identify

The simple answer to this question is that brains are made of carbon, hydrogen, oxygen, calcium, nitrogen, and a whole lot of other elements, just like the rest of our bodies. The more complex answer goes into how these elements are joined together into molecules and the structures these molecules make, and when you really go into the nitty-gritty, we talk about biochemical reactions and electricity.

When you pick up a fresh brain you'll find it has a pretty weird consistency. If you squeeze a brain in your hand, it turns into mush very quickly. It is pink and white in colour. That is the red grey matter, which is made up of the cell bodies and dendrites of cells, and the white matter, which is a fat used to insulate axons connecting different parts of the brain. (The red part is called 'grey matter' because that is the colour it goes when preserved in the lab.)

Has anyone ever called you a fat head? They were more correct than they knew – and the fatter the better. Take out the water and your brain is more than 60 per cent fat. (You'll have to take out a lot of water though, as it makes up about 80 per cent of your brain). Fat is vital to the proper functioning of your brain and all the rest of your nervous system as well. You'll learn more about it in Chapter 7, because the fat you eat directly affects the fat in your head.

Your brain is not just one lump. It has many distinct parts and each part plays a role in the functioning of your body, and hundreds of parts together form you and your concept of 'self'. This chapter introduces some of the major parts to you and briefly describes their major functions. We start by looking at the cells and then move to some of the large bits you should know about to understand your brain. Chapter 2 tells you a bit about how all these brain parts work.

BRAIN CELLS

There are more cells in your brain than there are grains of sand on the beach. They are tiny.

Most brain cells are called glia (or glial cells). These specialised cells make up the bulk of the brain's cells at about 90 per cent. There are a number of different types of glia and their functions vary from some that look after the neurons (star shaped astrocytes) to those that wind sheets of a fat called myelin around the axons (the oligodendrocytes).

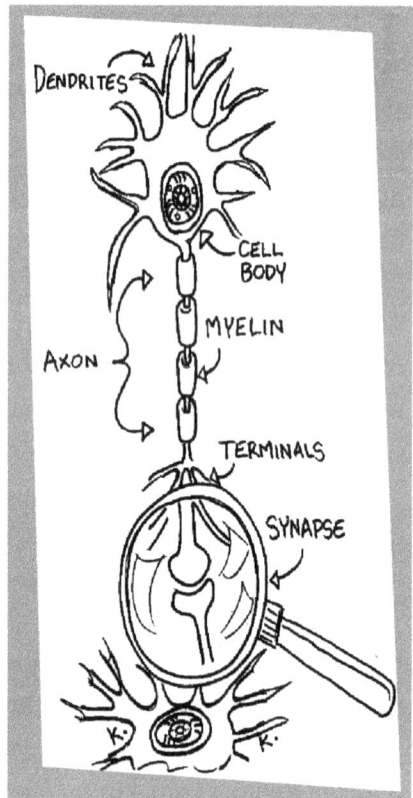

Figure 1: A neuron

But we're not going to look at glia here because it's the neurons (figure 1) that take up centre stage. Neurons are the 'thinkers'. They are the hard wiring of the nervous system that allows electrical and chemical messages to be spread around at lightning speed.

A neuron is made up of a cell body, which contains the nucleus, and extensions called dendrites and axons which end in terminals. There is usually only one axon, and it ranges in length from fractions of millimetres to the length of your body (brain to feet).

FUN FACT:
YOUR BRAIN USE 20%
OF ALL THE OXYGEN
AND ENERGY YOUR
BODY TAKES IN.

When we reach adulthood most people have about 100,000,000,000 neurons in their brains. That is one hundred billion! That sounds a lot but when we're born we have five times that number – more than the number of stars in the Milky Way Galaxy! We 'recycle' 400 billion cells in the first 20 years of our lives. Which ones? The neurons that are not used are taken out. Using a neuron strengthens it and makes it more likely to be used again. If you don't use it, the brain assumes you don't need it, so it is recycled.

The dendrites that extend from the cell body like branches of a tree are there to reach out to the terminal ends of other neurones, and they meet in a 'synaptic cleft' (see Chapter 2). The amazing thing about dendrites is that a single neuron can have more than 10,000 of them, all connecting with the terminals of other neurons. So if there are 100 billion neurons, just imagine how many synapses there are! I'll tell you in the next chapter.

MAJOR BRAIN PARTS

Neuroscientists have identified hundreds of distinct parts of the brain and more about them is discovered all the time, but let's look at the parts we can easily see during a brain dissection. I have presented them like a glossary so you can refer back to them during your reading to refresh your memory of their major functions.

The **Amygdala** is a nucleus of cells located at the base of the temporal lobe believed to be the source of emotions and emotional memory. It's the part involved in the flight or fight response – your immediate reaction to a threat.

The **Brain Stem** is found just above and connected to the spinal cord. It allows the brain to communicate with the spinal cord and peripheral nerves, and controls respiration, heart beat and swallowing among other things.

The **Cerebellum** (Latin for little brain) plays an important role in movement and control of your body. It's also involved in some cognitive functions such as attention and language, and probably in some emotional functions such as regulating fear and pleasure responses.

The **Cerebral Cortex** is the deeply folded outer layer of the cerebral hemispheres that is responsible for perception, awareness of emotion, planning, and conscious thought. It is a thin sheet of just six layers of neurons covering the cerebellum of a brain. If it was spread out and flattened it would be the size of a sheet of newspaper. This is where thinking takes place and memories are stored. The frontal cortex is often called the executive centre of the brain and it is the last part of the brain to mature during adolescence

The **Cerebral Hemispheres** are the two halves of the brain called the left and right hemispheres. They communicate well but the left usually is more involved with language (speaking, reading and writing) whilst the right likes music, and specialises in spatial abilities and face recognition.

FUN FACT.

THERE ARE MORE THAN 600 KILOMETRES OF BLOOD VESSELS IN YOUR BRAIN.

The **Cerebrum** is the bulk of the brain and is wrapped up by the cerebral cortex. It is divided into four lobes, called the frontal, occipital (at the back) the parietal (top) and temporal lobes (side). The cortex of the frontal lobes (the front divisions of the brain), is responsible for high level cognition (thinking) and judgement and this is where the conscious 'you' is. The parietal lobes deal with body awareness, orientation and movement. The temporal lobes (located on the lower part of the brain near the ears) are responsible for auditory processing and some aspects of memory. The occipital lobes at the back of the head deal with vision.

The **Corpus Callosum** is a large bundle of neurons that connect the hemispheres of the brain so that they can communicate with each other. Most women and girls have a larger corpus callosum than most boys and men.

The **Hippocampus**, near the centre of the brain, plays an important role in memory storage and retrieval and navigation and spatial memory. It's supposed to look like a sea horse (Hippocampus means sea horse in Greek).

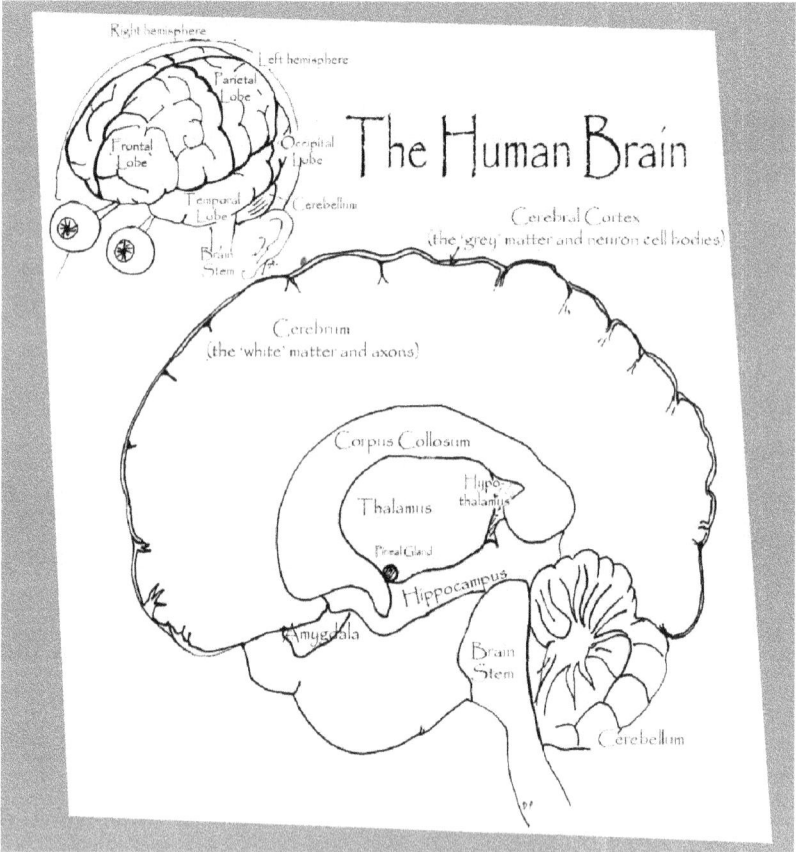

Figure 2: The Human Brain

The **Hypothalamus** controls body temperature, hunger, thirst, sex drive, aggressive behaviour, and the pleasure and stress responses.

The **Pineal Gland** is a gland that secretes the hormone melatonin, which is responsible for regulating your sleep patterns.

The **Pituitary Gland** is an endocrine gland about the size of a pea hanging off the bottom of the hypothalamus. It is considered a master gland and it secretes hormones regulating homeostasis (your body's default condition), including hormones that stimulate other glands.

The **Thalamus** is a pair of walnut sized balls of neurons which receive most of the information that comes in from your senses (touch, taste, vision, sound - but not smell) before sending the information to the appropriate parts of the brain. It is thus a relay station. It also has duties involved in screening out all the unwanted information you don't need and can ignore for now.

A MESSAGE TO YOUR TEACHERS

The brain parts listed above can be easily found during a brain dissection. Sheep or goat brains 'fit for human consumption' can be bought through your local butcher. An activity like a brain dissection is a prime example of Brain Compatible Education as it maximises sensory input and is a high interest learning experience. Brain dissections at school will never be forgotten – students will use the senses of sight, touch, smell and sound (but I suggest not taste). They will also have a good dose of emotional input I like to call the 'yuck factor', so the learning takes multiple pathways into the students' memories. Revisiting the dissection and rehearsing the learning through clay model making or artwork will ensure long term memories are created at higher levels.

A MESSAGE TO YOUR PARENTS

Parents want what's best for their kids. Educational experiences your teenagers have can open future doors we can't even imagine.

Your support for your children's education is crucial. They are at school for only about 13 per cent of the year, so although school may loom large in their lives, they are home and elsewhere for the vast majority of the time. Learning about the brain and how it works is an excellent way for parents to understand such things as the importance of rest, exercise, play and diet and the value of new experiences. It also gives you insights into how you can best support your kids when they are learning and developing effective study habits.

Chapter 2.

How Does it Work?

- -

IN THIS CHAPTER YOU WILL LEARN

✷ That nerve impulses are electric.

✷ Nerve impulses are also transmitted by chemicals through spaces called synapses.

- -

NEURONS

*N*eurons are awesome! From when we are little kids we are taught to be careful with electricity, and above all water and electricity don't mix, right? Wrong. Our whole nervous system is electric and works well in an environment that is 80% water! Messages are passed from one neuron to another in an *electrochemical* process using molecules that are electrically charged, and it is really fast. In the last Chapter you learned that there are about 100 billion neurons in an adult's brain. Each of those neurons is connected with perhaps 10,000 others giving you 1,000,000,000,000,000 connections called synapses. These numbers are so large they are mind boggling. Neurons are so small you can't see them without some pretty awesome technology. If the neurons in your brain were as big as a grain of rice, then your head would be bigger than the Earth!

The electricity we run on involves the rapid movement of positive and negative ions, or charged atoms. The ions that are most important for this are sodium ($Na+$), potassium ($K+$), calcium ($Ca++$), and chloride ($Cl-$), and a few negatively charged proteins which also have roles to play. How do they get charged? If you are in grade 8 or above you will, *of course*, remember from your science lessons that metal elements have extra electrons they can lose, which gives them more protons than electrons, hence positive charges. Chlorine, a non-metal, likes to grab the extra electrons and therefore gets a negative charge and becomes the chloride ion. So extra electrons equals a negative charge, fewer electrons equals a positive charge.

Like all cells, neurons are surrounded by semi-permeable membranes, which means they let some substances pass through but block others. In these membranes there are structures that act as little pumps. When a neuron is at rest these pumps move sodium ions from the inside of the cell to the outside and potassium ions the other direction, so concentrations are different on either side of the membrane. When the cell is resting there is a slow leak of potassium ions to the outside, but sodium ions are pretty much stuck. This creates an overall negative charge inside the cell. You can see that a difference like this will give the neuron some potential for action, or change, when needed. This is why it's called *resting potential* when it's at rest and *action potential* when it is not.

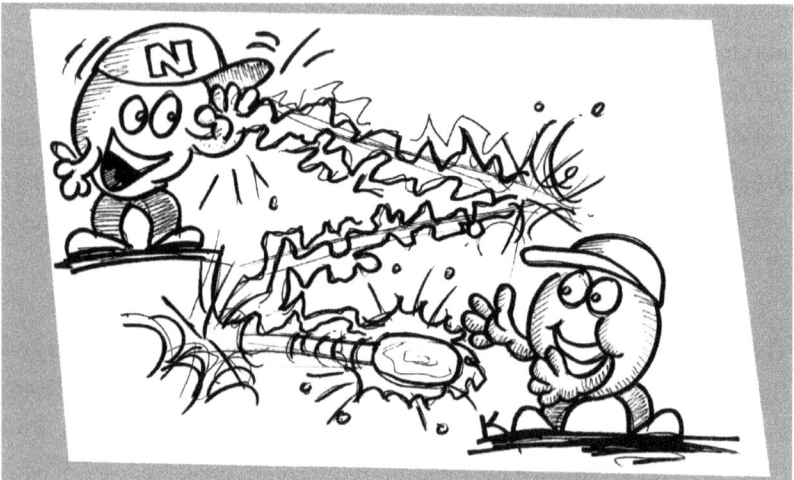

Scientists describe the work of a neuron as 'firing an impulse'. When a neuron fires as a result of a stimulus, an action potential moves from its dendrites, through the cell body and shoots off down the axon. This message transmission is simply the charged ions moving from one side of the membrane to the other to lower the difference in charge in an all-or-nothing event (there is no half-firing). After this, the ion pumps have to pump the ions in or out again to build up the charge and get back to the resting potential. (You can imagine how these pumps must burn energy to do their work, and that's one reason your brain gets hot after a lot of thinking, or you might wake up with a sweaty head after dreaming).

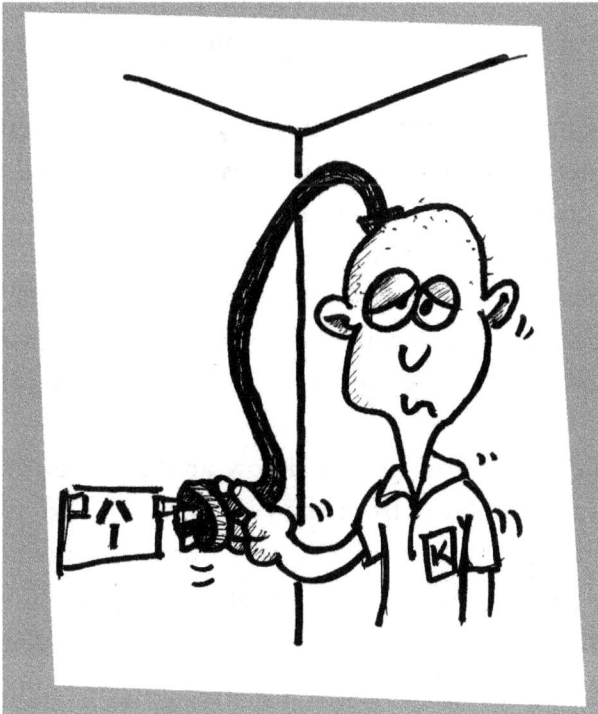

This is half of the neuron's work done – just a spike of electricity zapping down the axon to its terminals. The other half involves sending the message across the synapse to the next neuron. Synapses are gaps – neurons do not actually touch, but there is no little spark of electricity that zaps across this gap. Rather, the message now continues chemically.

FUN FACT:
YOUR BRAIN PRODUCES
ENOUGH ELECTRICITY
TO POWER A SMALL
LIGHT GLOBE – ABOUT
15-25 WATTS.

When the action potential arrives at the synapse from the axon, it triggers the release of chemicals called neurotransmitters into the synaptic cleft (the space between two neurons). The neurotransmitters are taken up by receptors in the next neuron and they change shape, which may excite the cell to release its own action potential. Then the first cell gathers up its neurotransmitters again ready for the next firing (which also burns up energy). All this can happen many times every second. The whole process may take only two milliseconds each time. There are about 60 different neurotransmitters, some of which you'll learn about in Section 3. Some are excitatory, which really get the next neurons going, but others are inhibitory and have a calming effect on the brain.

One other thing you need to know at this stage is how the neurons are insulated from the surrounding fluid and other cells. Why doesn't the electric current just go everywhere? The answer is a fat called myelin. Myelin is wrapped around the axons and it is essential for proper functioning. People with problems with their myelin may have the devastating disease called multiple sclerosis. The 'white matter' you see in the brain is essentially myelin. If you dissect a brain you can see masses of it running through the brain like rivers. These hold the axons of billions of neurons connecting to billions of others, creating the brain circuitry.

YOUR BRAIN

Phew! If you think that was complicated, consider this. Your neurons and their billions of connections make up your *self!* Everything you know and remember, how you react, your personality, likes and dislikes, your instinctive behaviours, your reading and evaluation of the information that comes from your sense organs and every thought you have, comes from the electric firing of these cells and those tiny puffs of chemicals in the synapses.

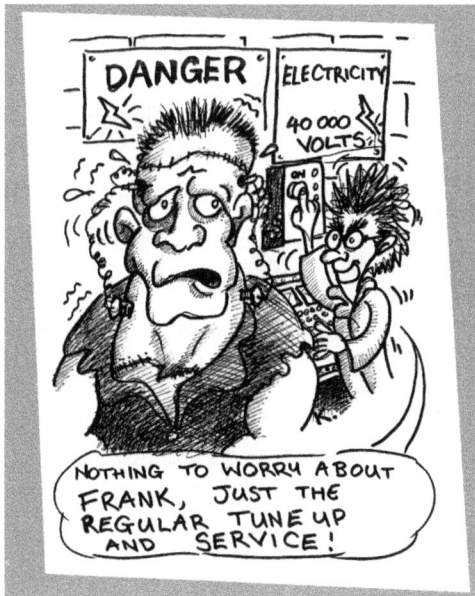

How does it all work? Biologist Lyall Watson said 'If the brain were so simple we could understand it, we would be so simple we couldn't'. So, it's not going to be easy, the biochemistry is complex and neuroscientists are still unravelling it. However, with the use of a simple model, we can at least make a start on understanding how the brain works.

The Information Processing Model (see figure 3) gives a clear pathway from the world (information our senses collect) to our actions (based on our learning) and therefore our effect back upon the world in a feedback circle.

There are giant textbooks, and thousands of papers written about this, but I am trying to put it all down in a few pages. So, for a brief introduction, here we go:

FUN FACT:
NERVE IMPULSES ARE ALSO TRANSMITTED BY CHEMICALS THROUGH SPACES CALLED SYNAPSES.

Firstly, don't think anymore of individual neurons. We have 100 billion of them for a reason. Think of networks of millions of interconnected neurons all working as one, firing together in the blink of an eye because a stimulus provided from the outside world is picked up by our senses (sight, hearing, touch, taste and smell). Senses measure *change* – if everything was the same colour and shade, without shape, you would not detect anything, until there was a change.

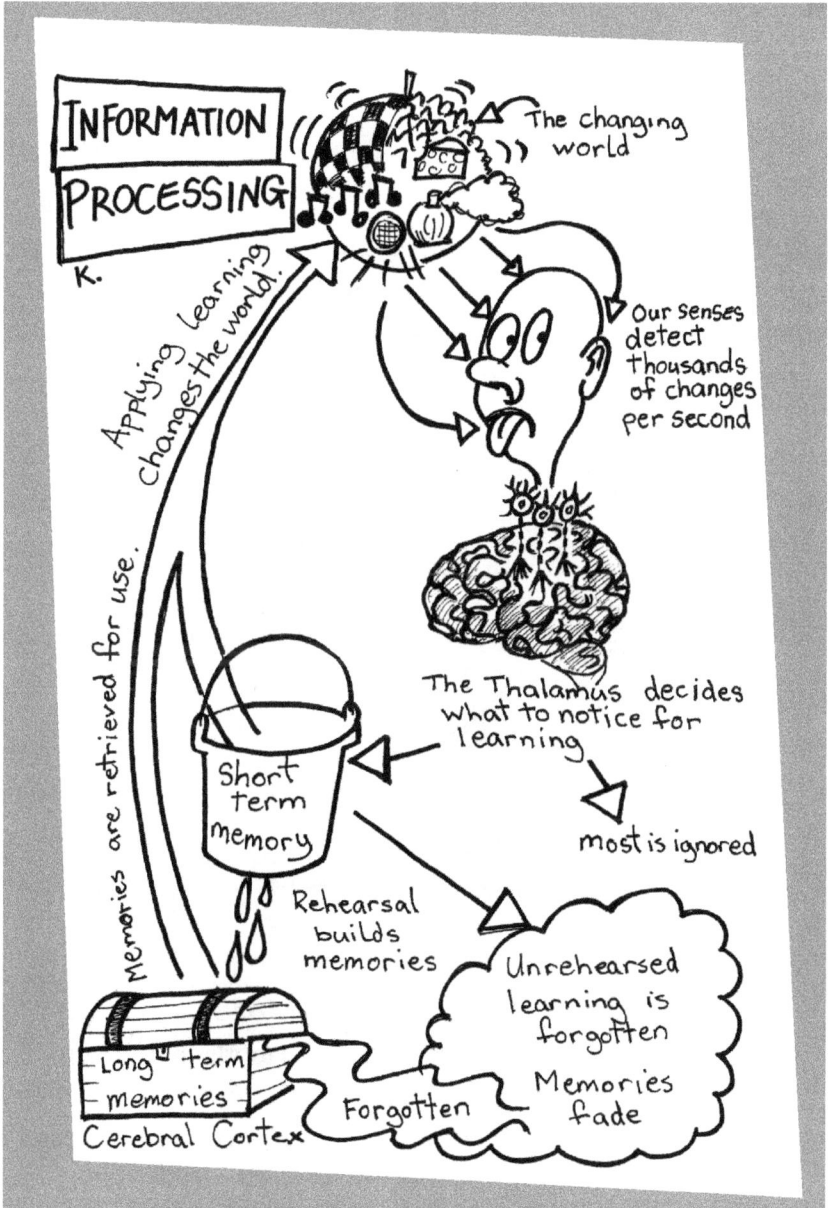

Figure 3: The Information Processing Model

Now imagine that after a network has fired there is some residual change in parts of the cells that lasts for a little while. This change is strengthened if the network fires again and again so it lasts longer. Then imagine that you can recreate the firing of the network at will. It may happen in exactly the same way as when the original stimulus caused it and therefore seem to recreate the effect. If we can recreate it like this without the original stimulus present, we can call that a memory. Our brains can then recall and compare this memory with others, sort them into groups, evaluate or re-synthesize them and use them to create mind images, which we call thoughts.

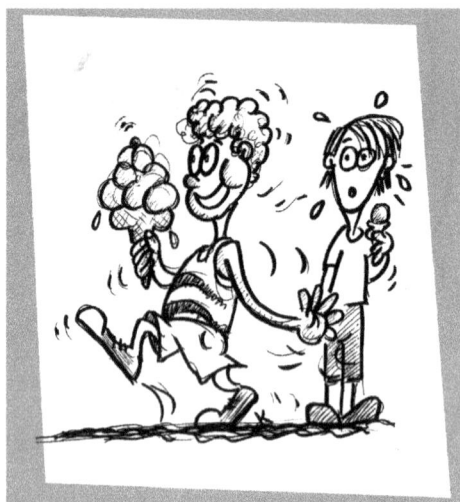

Here's a 'for instance': if I say the words *ice-cream*, your brain will fill in the context. You will have related memories pointing to the concept *ice-cream*, such as delicious, cold, creamy, white, cones, the freezer, and a million others that place ice cream into context. If you and I have similar memories of ice cream we will both know what we're talking about as we have the same concept and we can successfully communicate it. Some memories are more personal. If I said *Rickards* to you, you probably wouldn't think of ice-cream, but I and members of my family would, because the Rickards are our notoriously stingy ice-cream hogging cousins who dished out the tiniest servings of ice-cream to us when we were kids. What a shock it was, we Pughs were used to pigging out.

As you read in Chapter 1, different parts of the brain play different roles. Your senses are receiving thousands of discrete bits of information every second (as many as 40,000!), and there's no way you can pay attention to them all. Think of the feeling you have under your left foot right now. What's it touching? What does it feel like? A second ago you probably had no consciousness of those feelings, but they are always there. The touch receptors in your foot are sending the information direct to the thalamus in the middle of your brain. The thalamus decides whether or not to pay any attention, and ignores or dumps the information if it doesn't want it.

Some information from the senses buzzes around our cerebral cortex for fractions of a second (our sensory memory) but any information we want to pay attention to has to enter the *immediate memory*. If we want to learn it, it has to enter the *short term memory* and finally the *long term memory*, by being stored in various and multiple parts of the cortex. This is all done through firing the networks often enough to rehearse the new information and embedding changes into them so they are more likely to fire again in the same way, that is, be 'a memory'. We also develop 'pointers' to these memories that are spread across the brain which help us retrieve the memory. For example, cold and creamy sensations may point to the ice-cream memory (but perhaps also hair gel).

It's interesting to think that as learning creates *physical* changes to neurons a thought must also be physical – relying on connections between neurons.

The hippocampus is the major memory instigator and it is in contact with many areas of the cortex. The 'visual cortex' remembers colour, the 'auditory cortex' remembers sounds and other areas give you other clues to the shape and movement of things. You'll remember a parrot is coloured when you access your visual cortex and that it screeches when you use your auditory cortex to recall those memories. But it's even more complicated than that. Short term

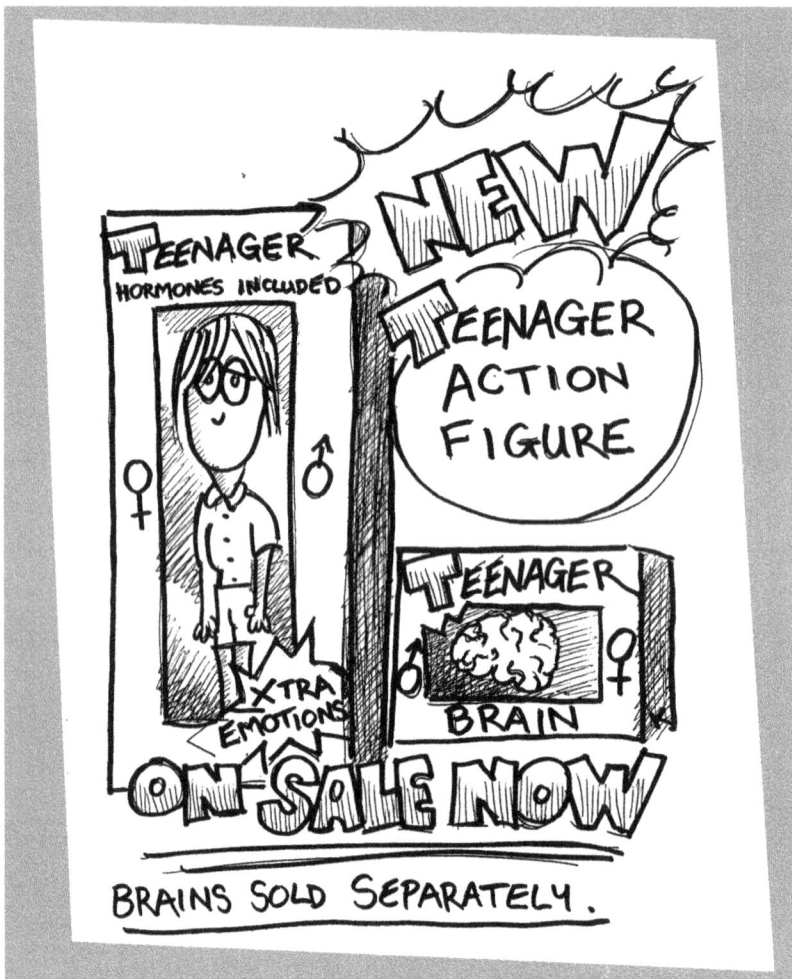

memory recall follows a path (called the Papez circuit), beginning at the hippocampus, it checks in on the amygdala to see if there are any emotions attached to the memory (e.g. 'yummy!'), zaps around the cortex collecting as much information as possible (e.g. cold, creamy, white, sweet), then returns to the hippocampus as, in our example, 'yummy ice cream'. If this circuit fires often enough it becomes a more stable memory, and it can then drop the hippocampus from the loop. It is then a long term memory.

You can easily see that if the circuit picks up information from multiple sources (for example, when a stimulus involves information about sight, sound, touch, taste and smell and contextual or historical memories connected to it), then it is likely to become a stronger memory because it uses so many parts of the brain. This is the basis of efficient teaching and learning. The more senses you use, and the more new information is given in context, the more you can learn. Also, what you already know is important to support new learning: try going into year 12 calculus lessons without knowing anything about maths and you'll see what I mean.

A MESSAGE TO YOUR TEACHERS

When most of us were at school the workings of the brain were still unfathomable. Slowly, really only over the last decade or two, neuroscientists have begun to understand how brains work and how we learn.

Today's teachers need to be aware of all this because we are charged with teaching brains, and much of what we have done in the classroom in the past has, unfortunately, not been brain friendly. Only those who were best suited to the delivery style efficiently achieved what their teachers were aiming to teach. Every brain is different. Brain based learning, or brain compatible education, is essential for our kids to reach their full potential. Today's kindergartners will be retiring about 2080, so we need to prepare them for... what? Everything and anything that may come their way! Many of them will have careers that haven't even been invented yet.

Many teachers need training in brain compatible education techniques. Schools need to access teacher trainers and resources to support their staff. Our knowledge of the brain is still in its toddlerhood, and our education model in 100 years might look very different to what it is now. We need to start moving towards that model now, and continue to adapt as we learn more about learning. The biggest change some can make, straight away, is to ditch wordy lectures and move to multi sensory learning experiences that increase the pathways for remembering the material. Go over the Information Processing Model again and refer to the reference list for resources by Jensen, Joseph, de Sousa and others to help you get started.

THE TOP 10
SUCCESSFUL BRAIN COMPATIBLE EDUCATION
STRATEGIES FOR STUDENTS AND TEACHERS

1. **EAT BRAIN FOOD**: protein and fruit in the morning, carbohydrates after school. And **EAT BREAKFAST!!**
2. **DRINK WATER** when thirsty, not sugary drinks.
3. **EXERCISE.** Move around at least every 15 – 20 minutes because it increases the oxygen content of blood and prevents the circulation 'bottle-necks' that come about from sitting too long.
4. **SLEEP** 8-9 hours every night. Avoid drugs.
5. Novelty is a major key to engagement. **Make learning memorable** through choice and self-directed projects but create class rituals to finish and begin each day.
6. Encourage students to learn how their brains actually learn.
7. Turn intellectual learning into applications as often as possible (=PRACTICE). Provide experiences that meet the needs and interests of the learner.
8. Incorporate regular, public rituals whenever students have achieved something special. Include celebrations, presentations, certificates, stickers and trophies. Demonstrate that learning is effortful but satisfying. Celebrate success.
9. Don't accept mediocrity, set high expectations. Treat all students as if they are highly capable. Use positive words rather than negative. Even the reading of negative words affects the emotional centres of the brain.
10. Tell stories and personal anecdotes with key messages about hope, resiliency, challenge and triumph embedded in them. Most people love personal stories (but especially tell the positive, uplifting type).

A MESSAGE TO YOUR PARENTS

When your kids were born they were not particularly clever. They had few memories, with very little myelin wrapping around their axons to enable efficient brain use and five times as many neurons as they'll end up with as adults. Neurons are recycled in a use-it-or-lose-it process that particularly accelerates during adolescence. Your teenagers are rewiring their brains and sorting out which neurons are to be kept and which ones broken up and recycled (this, in fact, continues to happen all our lives).

This is a major learning time. If your teens show interest in or aptitude for learning languages, sports, music, art, craft or anything else (that's positive) then the support you can give them now is the greatest opportunity to really contribute to brain growth. I suggest you don't waste money on expensive piano lessons if they hate them, but go all out if they really like them. Different brains have different interests. Some kids will excel in surfing, learning French, writing, painting, woodwork or countless other endeavours that other brains don't care about at all. Parents can nurture the unique and individual talents their children have for their lifelong advantage.

Section 2.

The Five Secrets in Preparing Your Brain for Learning

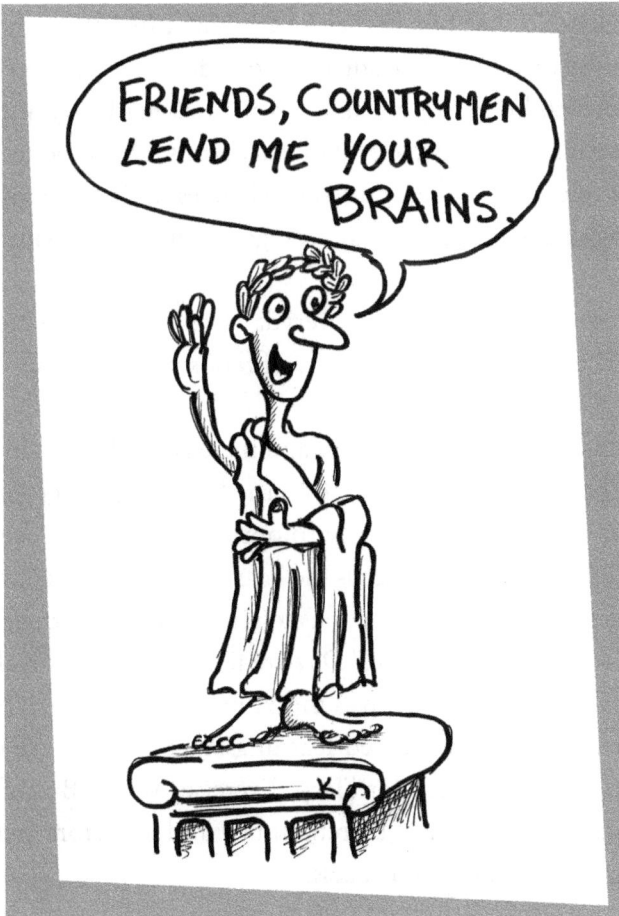

SEWBaD

Have enough **Sleep**
Have enough **Exercise**
Drink enough **Water**
Prioritize **Breakfast** and
Eat a healthy **Diet**

The rules of biochemistry are clear: we are what we eat. It is remarkable that our bodies and brains can accept enormous variations in their input and still function adequately. The variety and quality of diets humans are adapted to eat is extraordinary, and part of the reason for our success, in evolutionary terms. Other species, unable to adapt to changing diets caused by changes in their environments, have long since died out, or may soon go, as our own climate changes.

Not all inputs are equal – your everyday health, and even the length of your life, depend on the quality of foods you consume.

Much has been written about this and there is much you can do. For a start, though, if we concentrate on the following five ground level strategies we're well on the way to optimization. Why five? Brain compatible education concerns the 'learnability' of material. Five is a manageable chunk for most of us to remember easily, three or four is best. To help, *Breakfast and Diet* are linked, so there's really only four, but if you think of them as the *SEWBaD Secrets* you'll be using another excellent brain based learning strategy. Why SEWBaD? SEWBaD is an acronym for Sleep, Exercise, Water, Breakfast and Diet. Acronyms are easy to remember and therefore make the learning a more powerful process.

Chapter 3
Have Enough Sleep

· ·

IN THIS CHAPTER YOU WILL LEARN

* Why sleep is so important.
* How much sleep you really need.

· ·

We all think we know what sleep is. It's that time of the day when we become 'unconscious' and rest or dream, but why is it important and how much do we need? Experts differ in their conclusions.

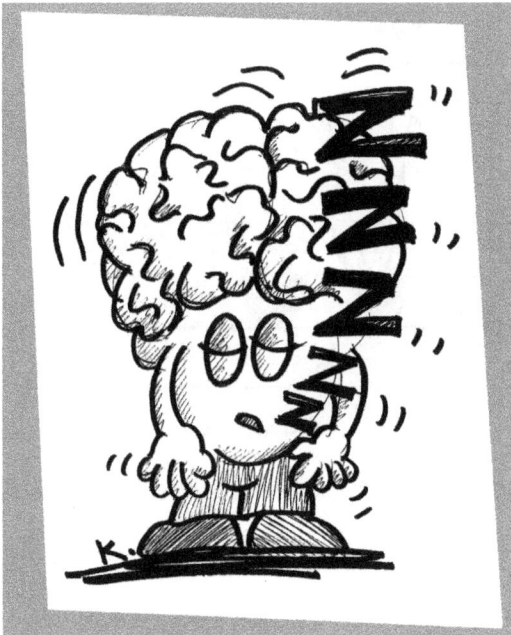

Some things are clear though: sleep occurs in cycles known as ultradian rhythms which are simply cycles between two types of sleep – REM and non-REM. REM stands for Rapid Eye Movement. It is called this because during this part of the cycle your eyes move rapidly (sleep scientists weren't particularly imaginative when they named it). REM sleep occurs in the last part of each 90-110 minute sleep cycle. It is during REM sleep that our brains organize and store some memories – particularly math concepts and language. The last stages of REM sleep, in the early morning before waking, are particularly vital.

Non-REM sleep is sleep when your eyes are *not* moving (aren't those sleep scientists clever!). Non-REM sleep is needed for rest and it allows us to be alert the next day. Some memories are formed during this time also.

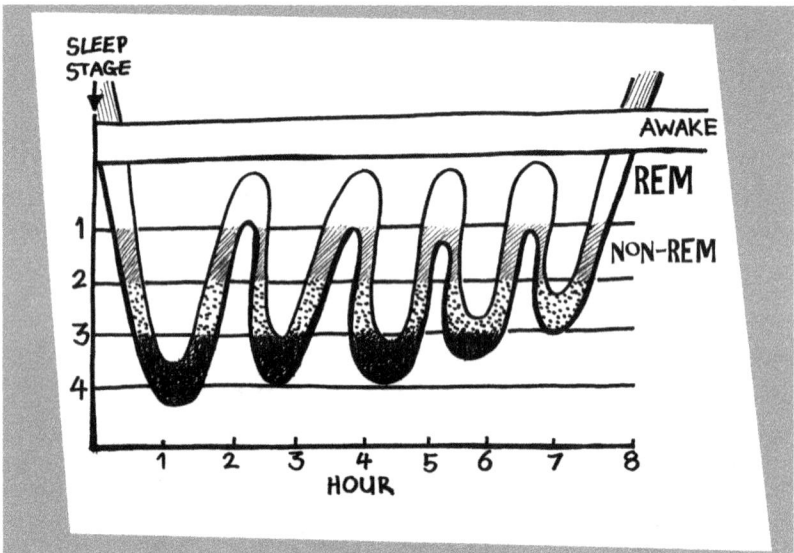

Figure 4: Stages of sleep. Dendrites make connections during sleep, retaining what has been learned during the day. REM sleep is particularly important for this. Non-REM sleep is important for rest.

Sleep scientists think that during sleep the day's learning is shifted from short term memory areas to more efficient storage systems in the brain.

The more you 'learn' during the day, the more sleep you need to remember it. Researchers are beginning to discover what effect a lost hour of sleep has on teenagers' brains. You may like to think about this in terms of your own sleep patterns: the researchers found that sleep problems cause permanent changes in brain structure and that some classic teenage behaviour (moodiness, depression, binge eating) may be sleep loss related.

Sleep loss can also affect which memories you get to keep, and the news here is not good. The emotional contexts of memories affect where it gets processed. The amygdala handles negative stimuli. The hippocampus handles positive, but it suffers more than the amygdala from sleep loss. The result is that sleep deprived people can fail to recall pleasant memories, but have no trouble remembering the gloomy. This may be a physical link to teenage depression.

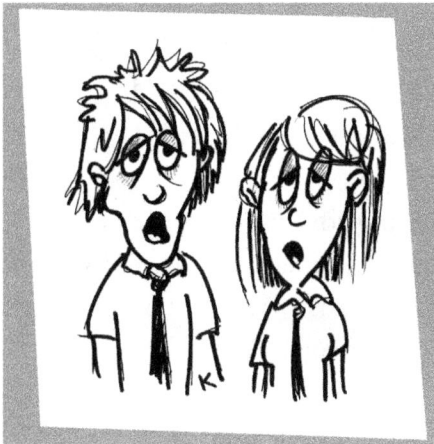

If we miss out on sleep, or interfere with sleep cycles, we can change the neuronal networking in the brain which can have a negative effect on academic potential and behaviour. If we miss out on sleep for too long, we die. Our society may have a problem because high school seniors already average an hour less sleep each night than their parents did at the same age. That's a whole night's sleep lost each week!

In two studies of nearly 10,000 students, teens who received *A* averages had fifteen minutes more sleep than those with *B* averages, and they had eleven minutes more than the *C* averages who had ten minutes more than the *D*s. So every fifteen minutes of sleep really does count.

FUN FACT:
SLEEP CAN SLIM YOU DOWN, PROBABLY BECAUSE SLEEP-DEPRIVED PEOPLE HAVE REDUCED LEVELS OF LEPTIN (THE CHEMICAL THAT MAKES YOU FEEL FULL) AND INCREASED LEVELS OF GHRELIN (THE HUNGER-STIMULATING HORMONE).

Some sleep scientists say that kids who miss an hour of sleep each night operate their brains at a cognitive level of about two years below where they should be. Grade ten students may operate as grade eights, so that makes the grade ten schoolwork that much harder.

If you are preparing for exams or tests by staying up late and cramming as much information into your short term memory as you can just before an exam, well, it's not the best way to learn. Your results will be better if you are wide awake doing the test.

Going without sleep for long periods affects you even more:

In 1965 the then seventeen year old Randy Gardner set the Guinness World Record for staying awake. He managed 264 hours (11 days) but had some disturbing psychological problems along the way – he had hallucinations by day four and developed short term memory problems and paranoia. He slept well after his record and managed to return to normal after a few days. The *Guinness Book of World Records* no longer reports attempts to stay awake because of the worry of causing serious harm. Now over 65 years old, Gardner told Gelf Magazine that he gets at least seven hours of sleep per night and his record attempt was the hardest thing he ever did

WHAT TO DO ABOUT SLEEP

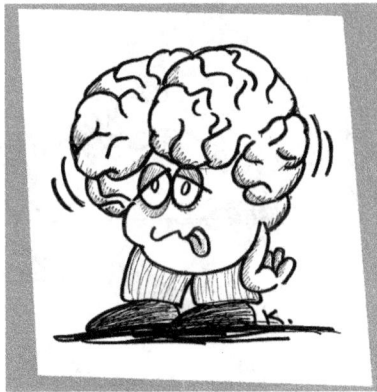

Do you feel you have enough sleep? Do you have a constant and calming sleep routine? There's no doubt we all need *sufficient* sleep – and that may mean 8 hours or more for many of us. This doesn't mean you can't have occasional nights out or watch late movies sometimes, because when we miss out on sleep like this we go into a 'sleep debt'. We pay off our sleep debts easy enough. In fact any sleep debt that builds up over the week can be paid off simply by sleeping in on weekends. Here's something to teach your parents if they complain about you 'wasting the day' lying in till noon on a Saturday. If you have a sleep debt this is the best, if not the only, way you can pay it off.

What about disturbances? Are you woken during the night? How can you ensure your sleep is as undisturbed as possible? There are lots of sleep disturbers, which we can call *sleep thieves*. Below is a list of some that affect some people and a table you can complete for your personal sleep thieves (from Joseph 2008). With an action plan, you can manage many of your sleep thieves better.

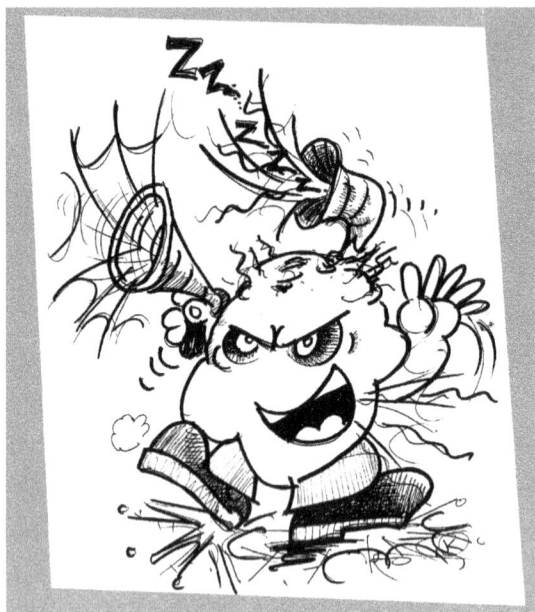

SLEEP THIEVES

School

During adolescence your body clock changes with hormones and teenagers may not get tired till after 11pm, and therefore get to sleep late. This means your REM periods may be cut short by school if you still have to get up early. This is one of the ironies of education. You may be waking up and going to school with your brain unprepared to learn well in the first two lessons or more. Sleep scientists say teenagers need later starting times than younger kids. Secondary schools that start after 9 am are more compatible with your brain. What time do you have to get up for school?

FUN FACT:
DOLPHINS ONLY SLEEP
HALF THEIR BRAIN
AT A TIME, AND THEY
ALWAYS HAVE ONE
EYE OPEN.

Movies/video games

Some researchers believe that stimulating DVDs and/or video games during the day provides strong competition for neuronal space and processing during REM sleep. Kids might learn the script of a film or cartoon before learning new material in the classroom, although you might not necessarily think this is a bad thing. I knew a boy once who was beginning to learn English as a second language so he wasn't very fluent. However, he could recite the entire script of *The Lion King* and could entertain us all for hours. What does this tell you about your own learning? Can you arrange your day so the more important things are given a competitive edge for processing by your brain during sleep?

We return to look at video games in a bit more detail in Chapter 10 because playing them too much can cause other problems.

Light

We are a diurnal species, which means that it is normal for us to sleep during the night, and be awake during the day. It should be no surprise then to find that to a large extent light controls sleep.

Light (especially blue) has direct effects on the pineal gland in the brain and its production of melatonin, the hormone that puts us to sleep. People who have flashing lights, computers or TVs running in their bedrooms, digital clocks etc, may have disturbed sleep without knowing it. Even the little red 'standby' light on many electrical items disturbs some people – I have seen some taped over in hotel rooms by guests who need the dark. How do these affect you? When you look around your bedroom can you see any light sources you don't need? What can you do about them?

Telephones and texting

Text messages at any time of the night from friends or spam may wake you up. Reading and answering them, or not, is a decision you make which can really affect your sleep. If this is a problem for you, what are you going to do about it? How would your friends react if you explain why you want to sleep and ask them to be more considerate? You could, perhaps, turn your phones to 'silent mode' when you're asleep.

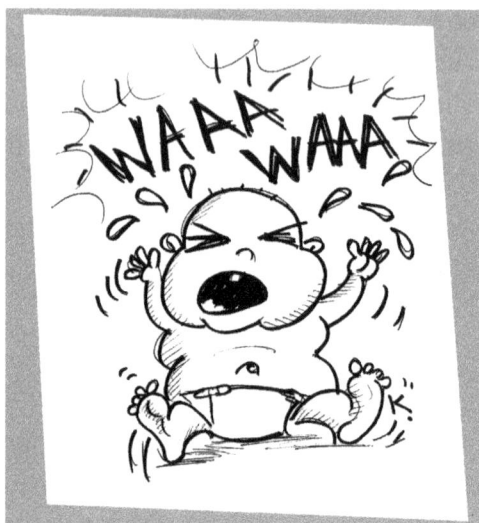

There is a time when we are all 'sleep thieves' for someone – are you considerate?

Your personal sleep thieves

Everyone has things that disturb their sleep. Can you identify your personal sleep thieves? What can you do to help yourself? On the next page you can make an action plan to 'arrest' them.

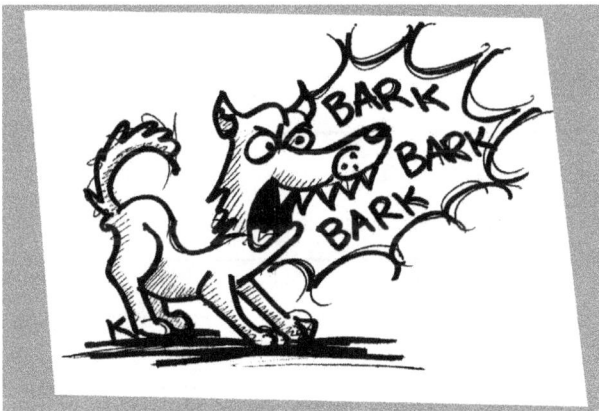

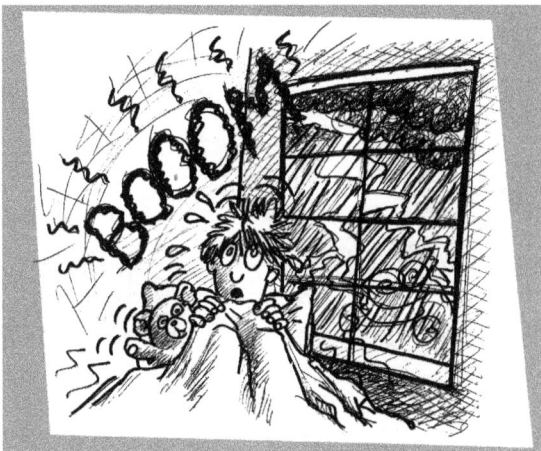

PERSONAL SLEEP THIEVES ACTION PLAN

What keeps you awake at night?	How can you get more Uninterrupted sleep?
1	
2	
3	
4	
5	

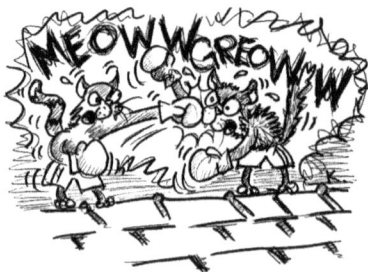

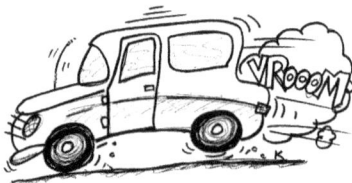

THINK ABOUT IT

✦ How many of the "Twelve Ways" relate to you?

Twelve ways that poor sleep can really hurt you.

1. Tiredness during class
2. Aggressive behaviour
3. Learning problems
4. Sports problems
5. Risk of skin problems
6. Risk of stunted growth
7. Risk of depression
8. Risk of being overweight
9. Clumsy behaviour
10. Social withdrawal
11. Motor vehicle accidents
12. Weakened immune system

A MESSAGE TO YOUR TEACHERS

Every teacher has had students start to fall asleep in their classes. It is not necessarily anything to do with how boring our teaching is (although the kids may disagree). Many of today's kids suffer from a continuous sleep debt, exacerbated by the fact we continue to insist they get up early for school, set them homework, and provide computers and the internet and all the other trappings of the modern world. Low points in classes for teens are usually early morning, before they are fully awake, or just after lunch, the 'siesta time' we demand they push through. (Under the influence of the hormone melatonin, twelve hours after the midpoint of the night's sleep our brains want another, shorter sleep).

Most teachers can probably point out those kids in their classes who are sleep deprived. They are likely to be the kids who either have their heads on their desks, or who are mucking about.

Behaviour might be an issue because in tired people the prefrontal cortex cannot metabolise glucose well enough. Their 'executive functioning' suffers, they have lower impulse control, and get distracted more easily. Many behaviour problems displayed by students disappear if they get enough sleep.

What time does your school start? In the US schools which altered start times to 8.30 am or later found dramatic results (maths and verbal SAT scores rose 15%). In another school they found teenage car accidents dropped 16% after later school starts. If you consider accidents, sleep can affect whether you live or die. In a school in Queensland, they had brought the start times *forward* to fit in with bus schedules. They went from a peaceful learning institution to a battle-ground in a few short weeks and then couldn't change it back because the kids had gone out and got afternoon jobs.

A MESSAGE TO YOUR PARENTS

Did you experience that 'fogginess' a new parent gets with disturbed sleep *every* night whilst your babies were still young? Did you notice becoming more forgetful? Searching for the car keys more often? Were you forgetting names, appointments etc? The time our children are babies is a time of unavoidable sleep loss. If this happened, you have an understanding of what some of our teenagers are going through today. The trouble is to them it may feel normal.

Sleep loss in our children may also be linked to the increasing level of childhood obesity. On average, children who sleep less are fatter than those who get their full nine or ten hours of sleep. In fact kids who get less than eight hours sleep per night are 300% more likely to be obese than others. Researchers, at the University of Texas, say your chances of becoming obese rise 80% with each hour of lost sleep. This may be because sleep loss increases the level of the hormone ghrelin which signals hunger, and lowers leptin, which decreases appetite. It also raises cortisol, the stress hormone, which has a role in making body fat as well. In one study, researchers at the University of Michigan discovered that 25% of kids diagnosed with Attention Deficit and Hyperactivity Disorder (ADHD) were actually sleep deprived and once their sleep issues were solved the symptoms of ADHD disappeared. Dr Leonard Sax describes the over prescription of ADHD medicines as one of the root causes of a large number of American youths suffering low motivation problems. Perhaps doctors and parents need to think about this before they start administering drugs to 'normalise' their kids.

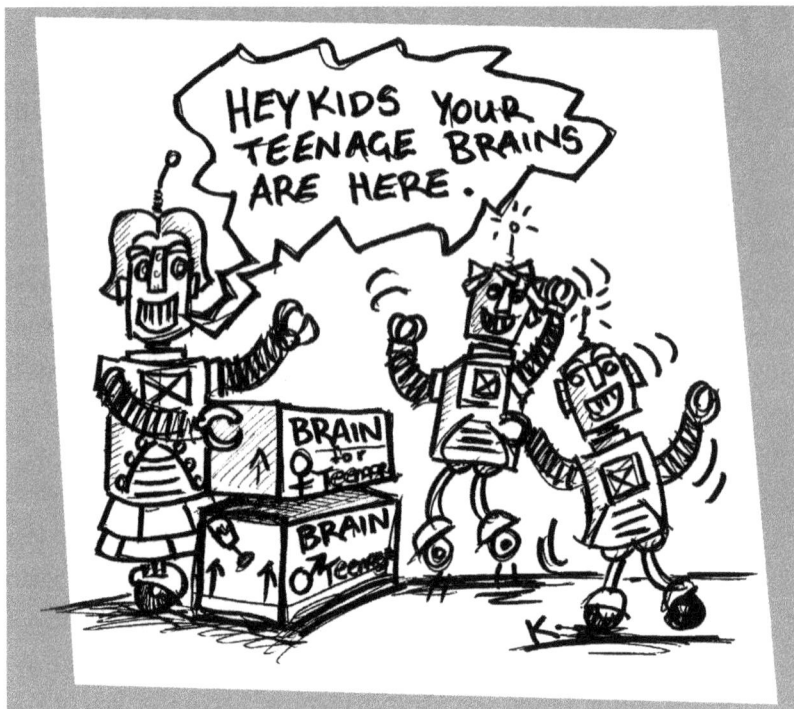

Chapter 4

Get Enough Exercise

· ·

IN THIS CHAPTER YOU WILL LEARN

✴ The importance of exercise to your brain
✴ That mental activity in the brain works just like physical activity in the body

· ·

What do you want to do when you leave school? There are professions and careers out there you will find challenging and rewarding, and others that might bore you silly. If you have an ambition, how will you achieve it over the next ten or fifteen years? Will you be fit and healthy enough to get the most out of it, and your life?

Many jobs, like much of school time, keep you sitting still all day and, even if you are doing what you love most, a sedentary life like this will affect you.

The shape of your body will reflect your lifestyle. Look around you at the successful and healthy adults who are in your life, on TV, or the movies. Who would you most like to be like when you are their age? What do you have to do to get there? You can bet that whatever their professions, if they are healthy and fit, then they are doing something about it to maintain fitness. They are exercising!

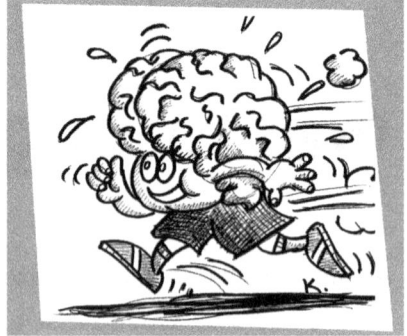

Physical exercise not only keeps your body fit, it is a healthy brain strategy. In fact getting regular physical exercise is a no-brainer for healthy mind *and* body.

How exercise affects the brain

When you exercise, your heart rate goes up to pump more blood around to get oxygen to your muscles. So it also passes through the brain at a faster rate.

Here's an idea. Stop reading right now, stand up and do ten star jumps. I'll wait......

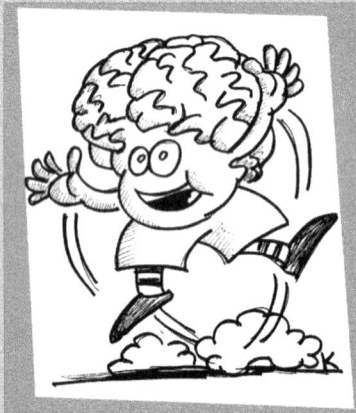

Done that? How do you feel? You have just raised your pulse rate through physical exercise, and more blood is flowing through your brain giving it more food and oxygen. Your brain is now ready to work hard again. Also, if you are reading this book in the library or a coffee shop, people might be looking at you strangely.

Increasing the blood flow during exercise increases the glucose and oxygen supply to the brain. Food supplies the energy and building blocks required by the cells for efficient functioning and growth – a process that produces toxic waste.

One of the functions of oxygen is that it grabs the toxic 'free radical' electrons produced in cellular chemistry and gets them out of the system as part of carbon dioxide molecules.

Our brains learn and grow because we interact with the world. Physical activity and mental activity have a direct influence on the brain's structure and function, and both can be improved through exercise.

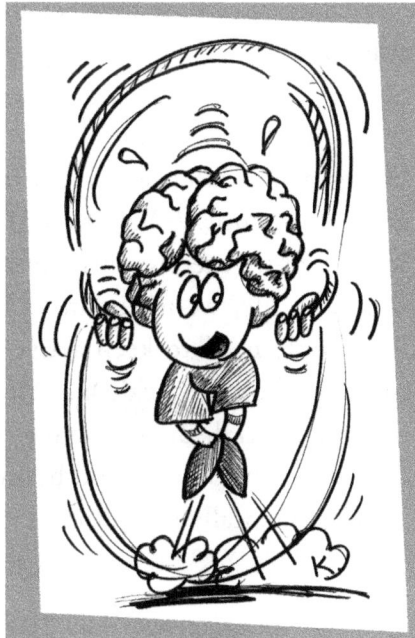

Doctors say that everyone, including you, should get 20 – 30 or more minutes of physical exercise each day, just for healthy body function. And what do you do after exercise? If you are like most people you will have a rest (maybe even a shower).

FUN FACT:
EXERCISE AUTOMATICALLY
GIVES YOU A BOOST IN
SEROTONIN.
THAT'S GOOD—THAT'S THE
HORMONE THAT MAKES
YOU FEEL GREAT.

Neuroscientists say we need mental exercise every day as well. Mental exercise means using your brain: learning something new, solving a problem, having a conversation and discussing something that stretches your understanding. Just like physical exercise your brain then needs a rest. Brain rest actually improves learning – a break every 30 minutes while studying will help you remember. Physical exercise and mental exercise together also protect against age-related cognitive decline.

I like the analogy of the brain as a muscle. It's been shown that grey matter becomes denser after learning a new skill – like a muscle, and it shrinks (or *atrophies*) after a while if it's not used, also just like a muscle. If we exercise this 'muscle' early on, and challenge it throughout life, we maintain its fitness. It is well known that older people need to keep active minds and they can learn a language, play bridge, or do anything else to prevent their brains going into neutral. Bingo playing by elderly people in England has been shown to be a good brain exercise. Bingo players remained more mentally sharp than the non-players, in one study.

Reading, it seems, is also good for your health. In Chicago they found that the reading habits of the under eighteen year olds were a key predictor of their cognitive abilities later in life.

Note that TV watching is *not* a brain exercise but you can watch TV as a brain rest activity for its entertainment value. Just don't go overboard. Scientists have discovered that many kids who watch too much TV, hours and hours of it each day, have a *lower intelligence* than more active kids.

Walking is an excellent brain exercise, as well as a highly physical exercise. Walking is not strenuous, but it increases blood circulation and therefore oxygen and glucose supplies to the brain. Studies show that cerebral blood vessels actually grow after exercise. If you're in the position to walk (or ride your bike) to school, then that is one of the best things you can do for your health.

Your brain is in a continual process of adapting and 'rewiring' itself. Even when we're old, we can grow new neurons. Doctors say that many age-related losses in memory come from inactivity and a lack of mental stimulation. This means *use it or lose it*, and there's no better time to start using it than right now.

Here's a brain exercise you can start with. Change hands! Whatever you're doing right now, change and use your other hand. It's hard – computer mouse movements, page turning, teeth brushing, your brain is so used to doing them the same way there's no challenge anymore.

Lawrence Katz, a neurobiologist at Duke University uses the term *neurobics* for this sort of exercise. It means doing normal everyday things a different way to exercise the brain – everything from travelling, to dressing or bathing with your eyes closed, or communicating without words for an entire soccer game. And you can try combining your senses – try listening to rain whilst smelling flowers or tapping your fingers.

You can think strong too. In Cleveland, scientists found that if you think about making a muscle strong through imaginative movement, after a few sessions, it actually increases in strength. In one experiment, people improved the strength of their little fingers by as much as 35%, just by thought.

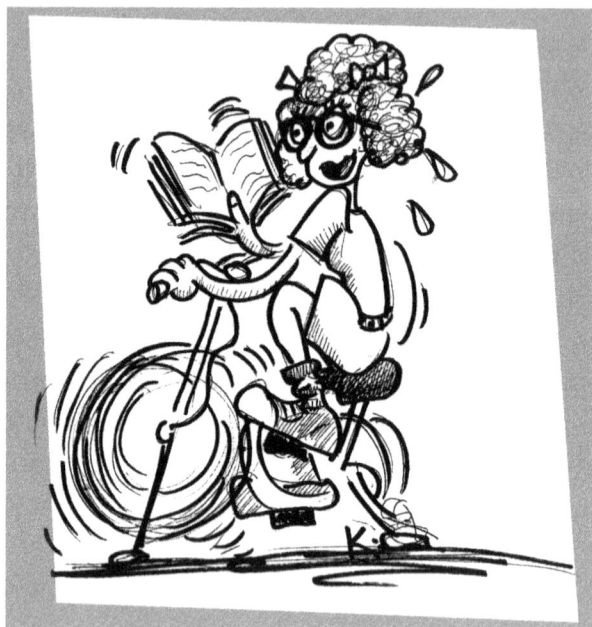

You can have a role here in the health of your parents or grandparents. In older people the risk of a stroke is more than halved even with just 20 minutes walking a day. Physical exercise has a protective effect on the brain and its mental processes, and may even help prevent Alzheimer's disease. A study of 5,000 men and women over 65 years of age, in Canada, found that sedentary individuals were twice as likely to develop Alzheimer's, compared to those with the highest levels of activity. So if you live close to old people, offer to walk with them. It would be good for you too.

Dr Michael Valenzuela says there are three keys to cognitive health – cognitive activity (learning new things), social activity (relating to others) and physical activity. All three are needed for healthy brain function. Now that you know this, if you've got sedentary family members, a little gentle teaching by you may do wonderful things for them.

Does the thought of regular exercise depress you? Don't worry because, as you'll learn in Chapter 9, exercise also decreases depression and helps the cognitive abilities of both males and females.

This is great food for thought. If we start life active and maintain regular mental and physical exercise throughout our lives, we're more likely to remain cognitively sharper than the couch potatoes next door.

THINK ABOUT IT

* Estimate how many minutes exercise you have most days:
* Do you think it is enough?
* What are you going to do about it?

A MESSAGE TO YOUR TEACHERS

Schools can help develop lifelong exercise habits in their students. Children need mentally and physically challenging exercise throughout their schooling. One follows the other, so in a crowded curriculum, schools which sideline physical subjects for pure academia do so at their peril. Schools are places where we train brains. Exercise is as much for the brain as the body.

Exercise changes in-class behaviour for the better too. Children who run around and play hard before class, are more likely to participate well in a class for up to several hours afterwards. Exercise also stimulates nerve growth, and affects the nervous system, by setting off the hormones serotonin and dopamine, which make us feel calm and happy. Perhaps it should be a prerequisite before any lesson. When children are calm and happy they learn more, as their entire nervous systems are working at a higher level.

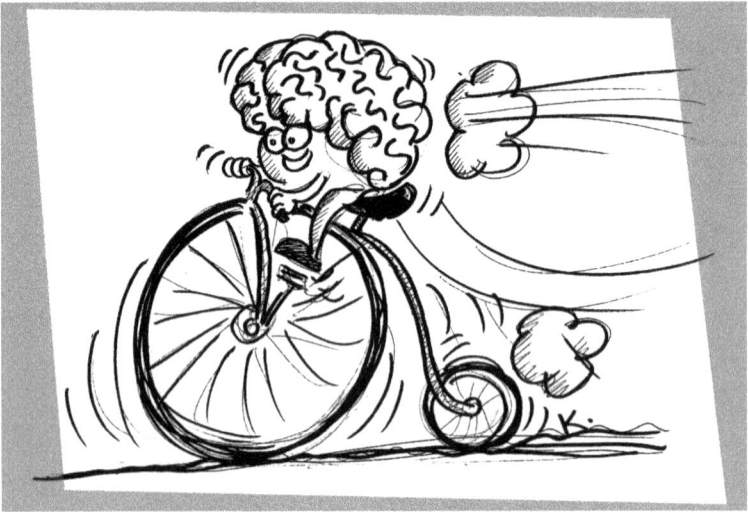

There are, of course, many factors other than exercise and the other four SEWBaD 'secrets' which come into play as a child goes through schooling. External factors such as home life, stress, abuse, and trauma can all have a negative effect on learning. However, exercise is critical. If we want learned, intelligent, adaptable and healthy children, exercise is one of the pillars upon which to build.

A MESSAGE TO YOUR PARENTS

Model good exercise habits to your children, but do so for your sake as well as theirs. As you approach middle age or older, physical and mental exercise is essential for you to maintain good cognitive health. Regular exercise is a tonic for the brain and evidence that mental and physical fitness delays the onset of degenerative diseases such as Alzheimer's disease, for example, is strong. I recommend Lawrence Katz's book on neurobics for ideas about exercising your brain. His neurobic exercises include simple things, like taking a different route to work, and shopping in a different supermarket than usual. Exercises like this help keep you sharp.

Chapter 5.

Drink Enough Water

. . . .

IN THIS CHAPTER YOU WILL LEARN

✳ Why we need to drink water.
✳ Why plain water is the best.

. . . .

Many modern schools now have policies where students are encouraged to have water bottles on their desks or handily available, but sometimes I despair of some kids understanding how important hydration is. When kids complain of a headache, the first question should be 'Are you drinking enough water?'

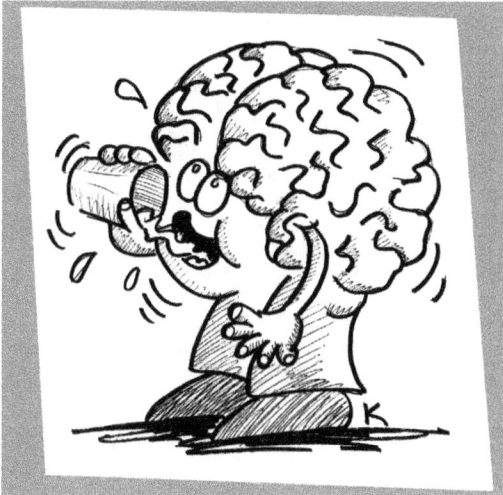

The science behind good hydration

There must be a very good reason why our bodies are 70% water, and our brains are up to 80% water. Among other things, we need water to think – if you start to dehydrate too much, your thinking starts to get fuzzy, and you may make poor decisions (think of the classic dying man in the desert seeing mirages).

Brains get 20% of the blood from every beat of the heart. Yet they only constitute about 2% of our body mass. This high investment in a single organ is important because it provides the glucose for energy and the water for essential neurological activities.

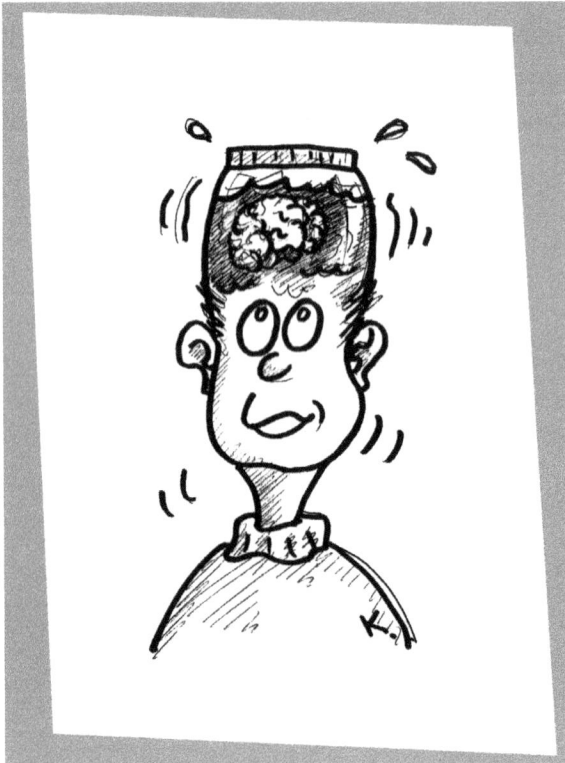

Poor hydration at any time affects how well your brain operates. This means it affects your learning ability. If you are slightly dehydrated you probably appear tired. You may have a headache or a reduced ability to concentrate. If you are usually like this, you might know no different, and think you feel normal. If you actually feel thirsty then your mental performance is already about 10% lower than before. Your performance will get worse as the degree of dehydration increases.

FUN FACT:
YOUR BRAIN IS NEARLY
80% WATER.
IF YOU LOSE 2% OF IT
THROUGH DEHYDRATION
YOUR ATTENTION, MEMORY
AND OTHER COGNITIVE
SKILLS ARE ALL AFFECTED.

You feel thirsty with a 1-2% drop in body weight due to water loss. In an average-sized teenage child this is about the same as a large glass of water. This could be the amount of water you lose during a sports lesson or recess time.

Drinking water immediately revitalizes the body and brain. It is in your best interest to replace any lost fluid. It is in your school's best interest to see that everyone remains well hydrated. Many teachers will encourage you to have a water bottle handy all the time, and to drink from it regularly. If your teacher doesn't encourage this, then perhaps you need to teach them how important it is.

Water is a brain booster and one of the secrets to ensuring your brain is ready to learn. Neurons work best at full hydration and stable pH, so you need to be well hydrated to maximize your learning potential. Drinking water regularly, throughout the day, will make you a better learner, but how much do you need?

How much water to we need to drink?

FUN FACT:
DRINKING A CUP OR
TWO OF PLAIN WATER
DURING AN EXAM
WILL MAINTAIN BRAIN
HYDRATION AND MAY
MEAN EXTRA MARKS
IN THE TEST.

Some 'experts' recommend eight glasses of water each day depending on your age, but this sort of quantitative advice seem to be going out of favour. Basically you need about 50% more water than you lose through sweating and breathing, as this allows a dilute urine and healthier waste management. In fact urine colour may be the best indicator. Learn to recognize when your urine is about the colour of pale straw, odourless and plentiful. If it's deep yellow, cloudy and smelly, or you don't pee at all, you are not drinking enough.

Alas, as with many things, there is a dark side you need to hear about. Drinking too much water can also be dangerous, as over-hydration causes a sodium imbalance that can be fatal – so don't go silly or drink more than you feel is right.

THINK ABOUT IT

✳ Estimate how many glasses of water (not juice or sugary drinks) you have drunk today already.

A MESSAGE TO YOUR TEACHERS

Most schools already provide easily accessible water to children all day and many allow water bottles on the desk or on a side table. This is particularly common in primary schools, where kids use the same classrooms all day. You may need to be a little more creative in high schools to ensure proper hydration of your students. And be consistent – water is for every day, not just during exams or sports events.

Schools can send a letter to parents explaining the health and learning benefits of having water freely available during the school day, and encourage them to provide individual water bottles the kids themselves can take responsibility for. You need to encourage students to drink *water*, not sweet soda or fruit juices. The brain accepts a sweet drink as a food rather than water, so it probably takes longer for the water to be of benefit and the sugar intake is unnecessary and an unhealthy option anyway.

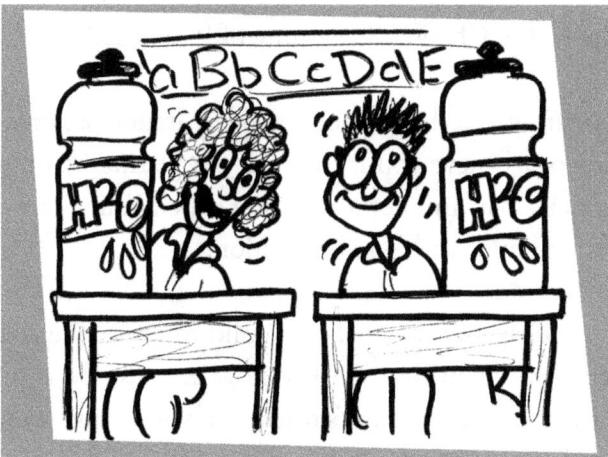

School programs should teach students about water and how important it is in their bodies. Remember, not everyone has read this book. Students may need to be taught explicitly of the need to check the colour and smell of their urine – dark yellow and smelly is not good.

A MESSAGE TO YOUR PARENTS

Parenting is a never-ending job. Knowledge is one key to making it easier and reading this book will help you understand the science of the importance of water to your child's learning. You need to encourage your child to drink clean water regularly. Give them water bottles to use at school and make sure they use water for hydration, rather than fizzy sugar drinks, milk, tea or coffee. It'll save you money too. A note about water bottles: you need to be aware that reusing some plastic water bottles, especially when using hot or cold liquids (or freezing them) may introduce hormone-like chemicals into the liquid that could have profound effects on our children. (See the parent message at the end of Chapter 7, warning of PET plastic use).

Importantly, you should model good hydration patterns yourself. Kids won't believe you if they see you getting by on ten cups of coffee a day and never drinking water. Your brain will also function better with good hydration.

You can help by teaching your child to check the colour and smell of their urine – dark yellow and smelly is not good. Lastly, talk to your school's teachers if you believe hydration is a problem during school time.

Chapter 6
Prioritize Breakfast

· ·

IN THIS CHAPTER YOU WILL LEARN

* Why breakfast is so important.
* The effect skipping breakfast may be having on your behaviour and your grades.

· ·

Breakfast is so important for brain function that it earns its own chapter in this book, even though it is a part of your diet (see Chapter 7). Breakfast provides us with the fuel for the upcoming day. Without it, we are relying on yesterday's leftovers, or breaking down body reserves. If you are working at school and learning new things, it is less efficient to be running your brain on the 'reserve tank' of energy. Breakfast gives you the blood sugar your brain needs for smooth cognitive functioning.

Many people skip breakfast regularly. When I ask groups of teenagers and school teachers how many have not had breakfast, I usually get about half raising their hands. People often use excuses like 'no time', 'nothing to eat' or 'I don't feel like eating until 10 o'clock'. Well, let me try and convince you to change your habits:

The science behind a good breakfast

When thinking about what you can eat for breakfast to best help your brain, it's going to be helpful if you understand how much

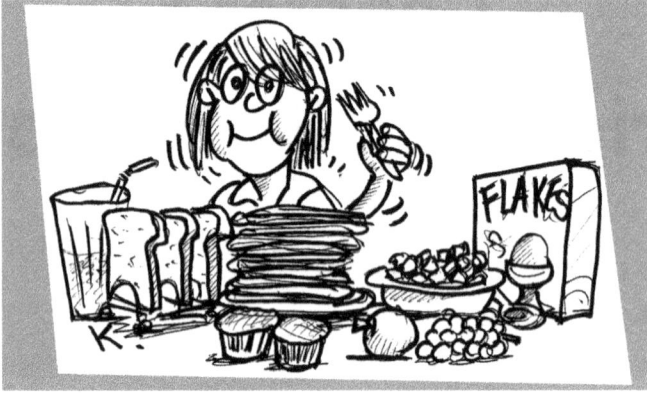

carbohydrate a food has, how easy it is to break it down into blood sugar, and whether it will give you a brief burst of energy followed by a slump (that may leave you craving more food, or sleep), or give you a sustained energy level that lasts for hours.

FUN FACT: PEOPLE WHO EAT HEALTHY BREAKFASTS ARE MORE LIKELY TO BE SLIM, BECAUSE THEY ARE LESS LIKELY TO SNACK DURING THE DAY.

There is a number system which measures the 'sugar hit' a food gives you called the Glycemic Index (GI). When you eat a carbohydrate, it is quickly digested and becomes blood sugar (sugar dissolved in your blood in a form it can be absorbed by cells). A high GI simply tells you how rapidly a particular carbohydrate turns into blood sugar. On a chart, a high GI food will trigger a dramatic spike in blood sugar, but a low GI food will show a slower longer lasting response. (A GI of 70 or more is high and a GI of 55 or less is low. Pure glucose has a GI of 100). Think about this for a moment: which are you likely to need – the rapid response or the slow one?

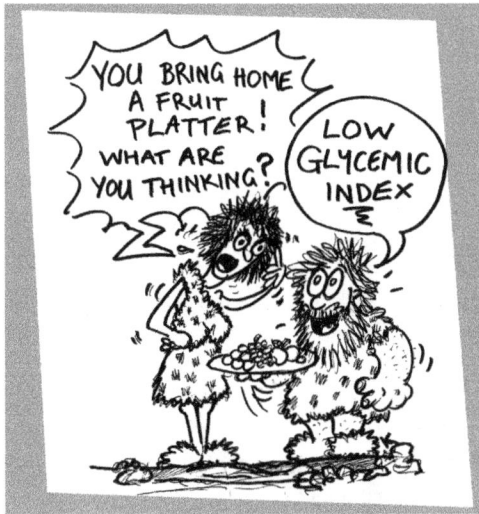

Another scale called the Glycemic Load (GL) is more useful if you are comparing foods. The GL tells you how much carbohydrate is in a food. To avoid a high carbohydrate diet most of your food should have a low GL, less than ten.

So what does this mean to your breakfast? Well, to keep blood sugar at a steady level for the brain for an extended period, we need to avoid the spikes of the sugar hit. Obviously, not all breakfasts are the same, and it is clear eating some foods may be worse than not eating at all. Chapter 7 warns you about having too much sugar and the wrong type of fats in your diet. If you eat, for example, deep-fried sugar-donuts for breakfast, you get a spike in blood sugar lasting a few moments only, plus a blast of trans-fats, and not much else, except another step on the road to obesity. However, if you eat foods which will release energy slowly, you won't get hungry again quickly, which means you'll make it through to recess or even lunchtime without having to refuel, and you won't 'crash' as the spike ends and fall asleep in second lesson.

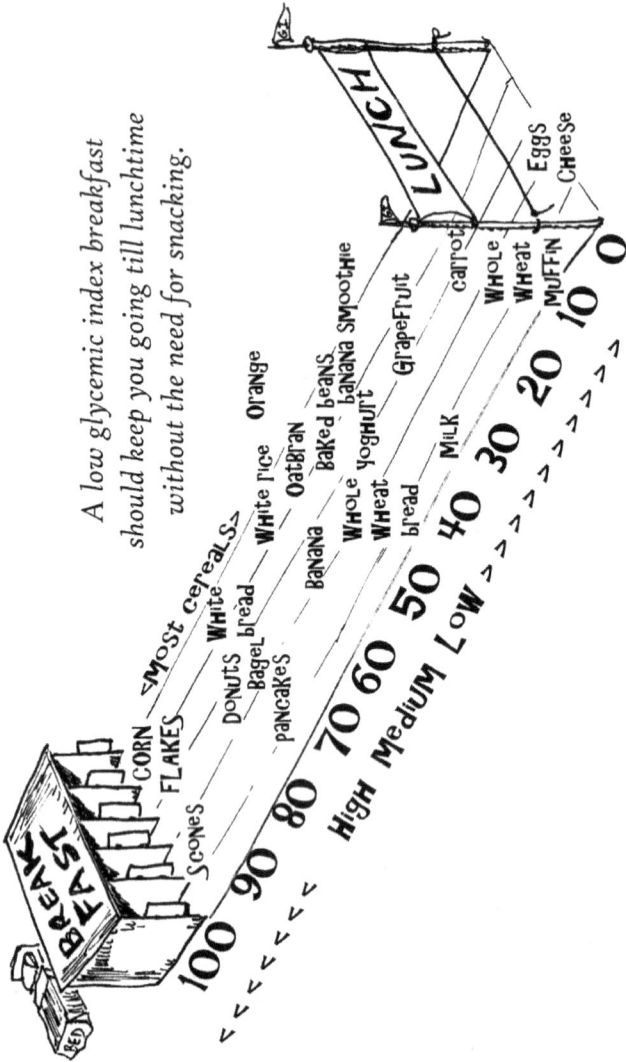

A low glycemic index breakfast should keep you going till lunchtime without the need for snacking.

LUNCH

Eggs
Cheese

Whole Wheat MUFF'N

carrot

Grapefruit

Whole Wheat bread

Whole yoghurt

Milk

Baked beans

banana smoothie

OatBran

Orange

White rice

Banana

Most cereals

White Bagel bread

Donuts

pancakes

CORN FLAKES

Scones

BREAKFAST

100 90 80 70 60 50 40 30 20 10 0

High Medium Low

Figure 5 The Glycemic Index race

The research on the effects of breakfast and student functioning seems pretty straight forward: *If you are someone who has a good breakfast you are a better student.*

Nutritionist Anne Nilsson says that a low GI aids the working of short term memory. You can concentrate better, and can manage more complex tasks. You are likely to be able to make it to lunch time comfortably, are more likely to eat a nutritious lunch, and less likely to overeat. You probably show better behaviour and learning, as you may be calmed by the process of eating a good breakfast, thereby lowering cortisol and other stress hormones, plus it's likely you have a better attitude towards schooling. You also get fibre, water and important nutrients like calcium, through your breakfasts and you are likely to have lower cholesterol levels, and fewer days off school sick, than your non-breakfast-eating classmates.

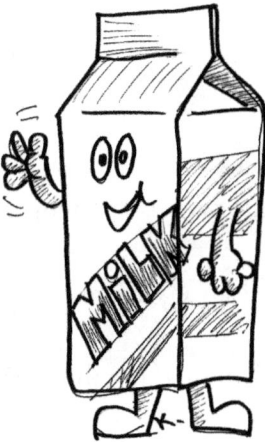

However for those who skip breakfast, or eat lots of sugar and the wrong type of fats, well, simply, you will be getting lower grades than you would otherwise. You will have an empty belly most of the morning and are likely to crave junk food. You are likely to be overweight and sluggish. If you don't believe me try an experiment – trial eating good breakfasts for a term and see if you notice any differences.

If you are overweight, or have a poor body image, skipping breakfast is *not* the way to lose weight. That extra body weight is probably there because of the *quality* of food, not necessarily the quantity. Eat well, with fruits, nuts, oats, eggs, and cheese, yoghurt etc, and your body will take care of itself.

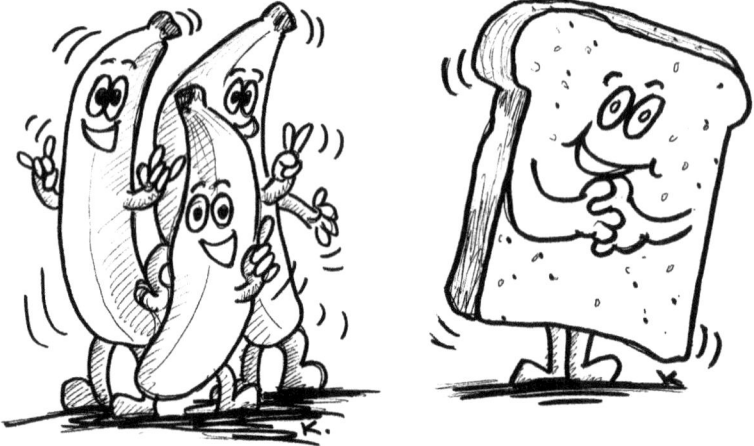

TRY THIS

* Eat breakfast every day for the next week
* Read the nutritional information on the packet of anything you eat.
* Note down the approximate amount of sugar you are eating at breakfast.
* Decide if this is a problem. Should you do anything about it?

THINK ABOUT IT

Are you a Breakfast Winner or Loser?

We live in enlightened times. A scan of the work of nutritionists and neuroscientists tells us how the brain obtains and uses the chemicals it needs for healthy function and the overwhelming importance of breakfast. Not just any breakfast however, as it is clear eating some foods may be worse than not eating at all.

We are breaking our fast at breakfast time. Breakfast provides us with the fuel for the upcoming day. Without it we are relying on yesterday's leftovers, or breaking down body reserves.

At school evidence for the value of breakfast is high. There are winners and losers. It's simple:

* Breakfast winners have nutritious breakfasts.
* Breakfast losers skip breakfast or eat lots of sugar and the wrong type of fats.
* Breakfast winners are better students. They concentrate better and can manage more complex tasks.
* Breakfast losers get lower grades.
* Breakfast losers have an empty belly and are likely to crave junk food during the morning.
* Breakfast losers are often overweight and sluggish.
* Breakfast winners can make it to lunch time comfortably and are more likely to eat a nutritious lunch and less likely to overeat.
* Breakfast winners eat complex carbohydrates and proteins in roughly equal amounts in terms of energy. (Carbohydrates alone can make you drowsy).
* Breakfast winners often have high calcium levels in their breakfasts (eg through dairy products) and show better behaviour and learning.
* Breakfast winners may be calmed by the process of eating a good breakfast, thereby lowering cortisol and other stress hormones.
* Breakfast winners often have a better attitude towards schooling.
* Breakfast winners also get fibre, water and other important nutrients through their breakfasts.
* Breakfast winners are likely to have lower cholesterol levels and fewer days off school sick.

A MESSAGE TO YOUR TEACHERS

I asked a group of 200 middle school students recently for a show of hands to the following questions: Who had breakfast this morning? Who went to bed last night after 11 pm? And who thinks they are among the group that gets in trouble most at school? You guessed it, the same kids kept their hands up. School behaviour and achievement is inextricably linked to the five 'secrets' I outline in this book. Happy schools, with well functioning students and teachers, can only run on good fuel and sufficient rest. (By the way, many of the teachers at this school had also skipped breakfast.)

Schools have a role not only in education of students but in what they offer at school canteens. It is worth making an audit of what is prepared and sold and how much junk is chosen over good food. School canteens need to avoid providing the high sugary junk.

Once I was a teacher on a small island. The community store was right beside the school and many students went to the store for a breakfast of soda drinks and chips at recess. The result: classroom behaviour after recess was markedly different, some of the kids were bouncing off the walls, but by lunchtime they were quiet and sleepy. Having a dramatic spike in blood sugar, that lasts for only a few minutes, is detrimental to classroom functioning as well as learning, though may be useful in 100m sprint races. The GL is a useful guide here and school canteens (or kids' lunch boxes) can be filled with foods of low-medium GL to provide sustaining levels of blood sugar.

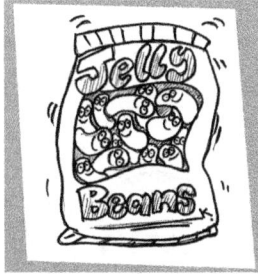

A MESSAGE TO YOUR PARENTS

Getting your teenagers to eat a sufficient and healthy breakfast may not be an easy thing to do. If they have read this Chapter they may understand why they need it, but in the morning rush, with tempers flaring or general just-out-of-bed grumpiness, it's easy to skip eating.

The work of parents seems never-ending but there are several things you need to ensure. Firstly, breakfast foods must be available. Secondly, check that your cooked foods, raw foods, cereals, breads and so on, are healthy, without a high sugar or trans-fat content.

Breakfasts take time, so plan ahead and make sure there is enough.

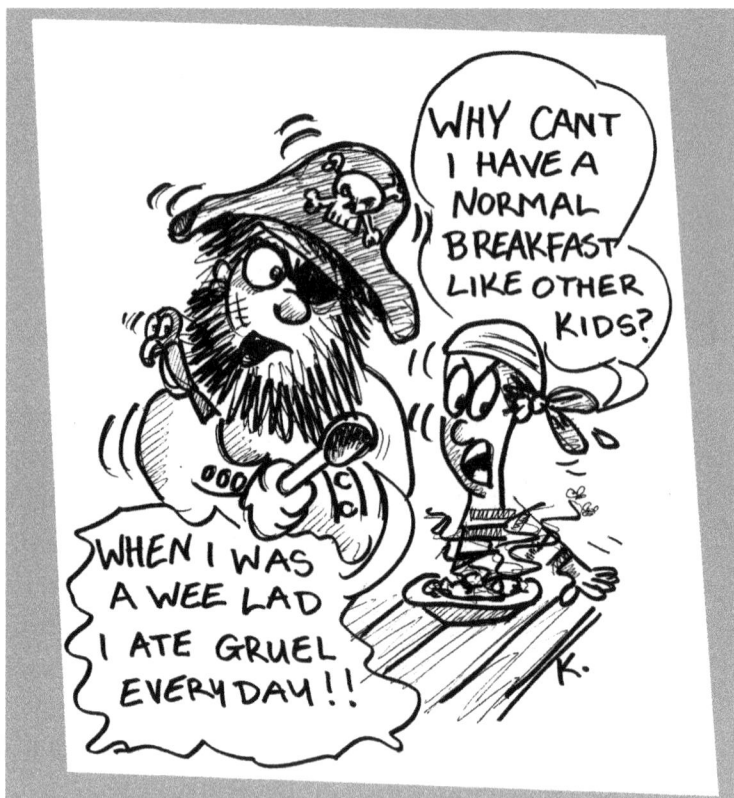

Chapter 7

Eat a Healthy Diet

. . . .

IN THIS CHAPTER YOU WILL LEARN

* The difference between different carbohydrates and how they affect your brain.
* That there are 'good' fats and 'bad' fats and what the differences are.

. . . .

Big Ron was one of those kids who could do anything. Really smart, even brilliant, particularly in manual arts: he could build anything. He left school early to seek his fortune in the mines of the Northern Territory of Australia. He worked 'out bush', making lots of money and eating at the daily barbeques put on by his company – the best beef steak, barbeque sauce and beer, as much as he wanted.

After a couple of months out bush, he says, he started to feel a bit sick. His head ached and his gums hurt, his breath stank, he felt weak and it was hard to get out of bed. So a mate drove him into town to see a doctor. He was told he had the beginnings of scurvy. *Scurvy*! The scourge of the old sailing ship days, responsible for thousands of sailors dying slow, lingering, and painful deaths in the 1600s and 1700s!

Scurvy is caused by a lack of vitamin C. You easily get vitamin C from eating fresh fruits and vegetables, but there is none in beef steaks. And it only takes around six weeks to develop if you don't get enough Vitamin C. Big Ron had a wakeup call he's never forgotten. He eats a much healthier diet now.

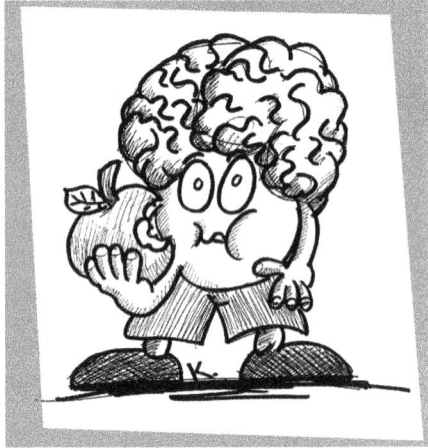

Diet is so important to our wellbeing that being aware of what we eat really can be a matter of life or death. The trouble is, an early death in 30 years time rather than 50 or 60 years seems so far removed for teenagers, it's easy to get into bad eating habits now. But healthy food cookbooks are available in their thousands. You probably already know what healthy food looks like, what junk food is, and the effects of a poor diet on your body. This Chapter, however, is about why you should watch your diet from your brain's point of view.

Think now about what you eat and drink. How much junk have you eaten today? Do you do this every day? Everything you need to build a healthy brain, except oxygen, must come from your food and drink. There's no other way.

A number of essential vitamins and minerals, essential fatty acids and essential amino acids (to make proteins) must come from your diet, that's why they're called 'essential'. If you miss out on them you run the risk of getting a 'deficiency disease' like scurvy, rickets (lack of vitamin D, calcium and phosphate), goitre (lack of iodine) or a

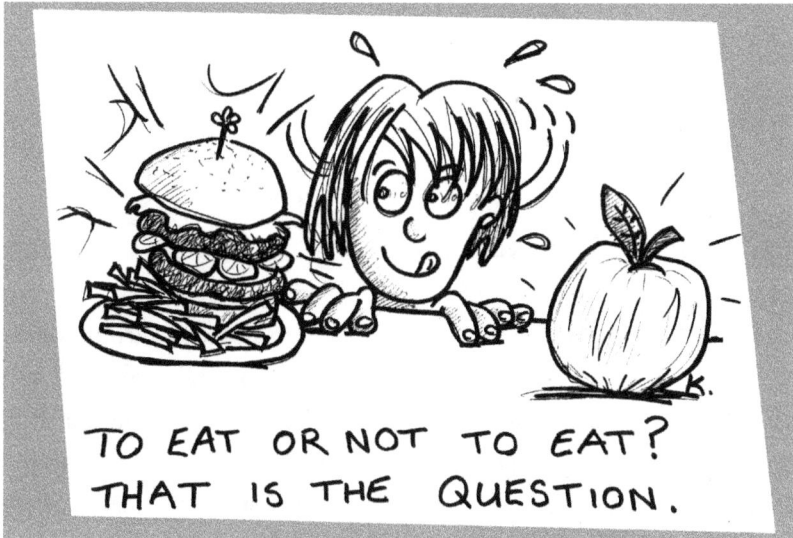

TO EAT OR NOT TO EAT?
THAT IS THE QUESTION.

whole host of others. By law, in most countries, food packaging must list what is inside the food. You should get used to reading this list. Note that ingredients are listed in descending order of percentage. So, if a list says 'sugar, flour ....' in that order, it means it contains more sugar than flour. And if sugar weighs 20 grams for every 100 grams of the food you're eating... well, you do the maths.

If your meals arrive wrapped in plastic, or straight from the microwave, after being flash frozen or deep fried, then you will already know you're eating poorly. I am not going to repeat the bad news here – your waist line is probably reminder enough, or soon will be, after you leave your teens. But as a brain education consultant, I only have more bad news for you. Junk food diets lead to junk brains. Neuroscientists say that on a junk food diet your IQ suffers, your intrinsic motivation sinks, you are more likely to be a couch potato than a Rhodes Scholar. As you get older, the risk of suffering memory loss is substantially higher. You could be heading towards diabetes, or insulin resistance or towards an early grave. Why is this?

The science of brain chemistry is complex but clearly building a quality brain requires quality building blocks. If you use substandard materials you get what you've paid for. The two major brain nutrients we will focus on in this Chapter are carbohydrates and fats.

Carbohydrates and your brain

The brain only uses one major fuel source, glucose, a carbohydrate. Glucose is what we call 'blood sugar'. Our brains need about a half cup of glucose a day (100 grams) to function properly. This is a large amount but it's easy to get. At some times of our lives, for example during pregnancy, or on a doctor's advice, we may need dietary supplements of essential brain nutrients, but the carbohydrate part of our diet is the one that will never require supplementing. Unfortunately, many of the junk foods we eat give us massive, unneeded, carbohydrate blasts.

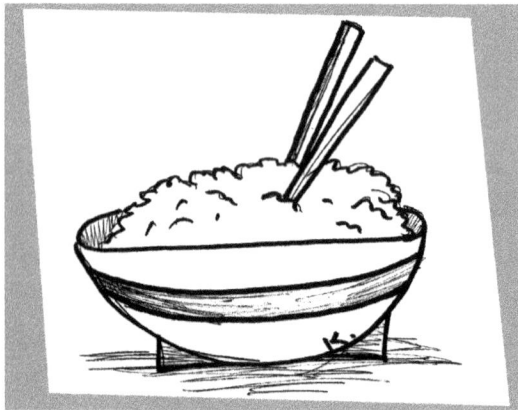

In fact, carbohydrates are so easy to come by in this day and age, that we all have too much. Our ancestors roamed the plains of Africa with the nearest convenience store millennia away, and in some seasons carbohydrates were undoubtedly scarce. But they survived anyhow, because humans evolved a remarkable ability to make all the 100 grams of glucose our brains require from the protein they ate every day. So we don't need to eat carbohydrates at all, as far as the brain is concerned.

We can store enough glucose as blood sugar to last about 24 hours. After that the body's survival mechanism is to break down our own protein 'stored' as muscle or in other organs. We evolved to eat a diet of fats and proteins; everything from grasshoppers to zebras, with occasional and limited carbohydrates thrown in. So it's no surprise to find that we can exist without donuts, French fries and Black Forest cakes. The brain is a sugar addict – but I stress, *we don't need to eat it*. In fact, our bodies give priority to the brain in times of shortages, or even starvation, because the muscles and the other organs can operate on a different fuel source for energy production: fat.

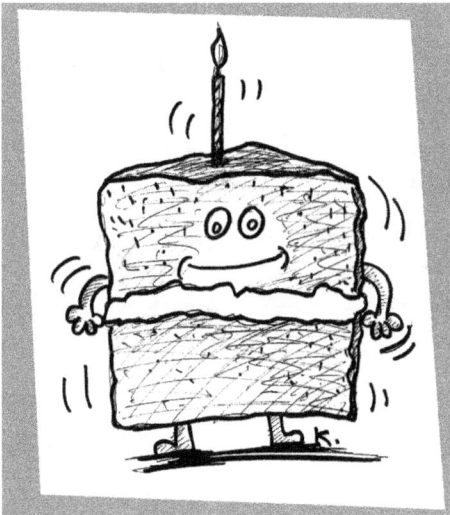

This leaves the glucose for the brain. Our bodies use the hormone *insulin* to control this. Insulin drives sugar and proteins into the cells so they can be used in their chemical processes. In periods of shortage, all cells except brain cells become temporarily insulin resistant, so the brain can continue to function normally.

The problem is with a high sugar diet, our brains are awash in a sea of blood sugar that we have not evolved to cope with. Too much blood sugar for too long can create insulin resistance in brain cells as well, and that's not good. As neurosurgeon, Dr Larry McCleary says, 'all the blood sugar in the world can't fuel a brain resistant to insulin'.

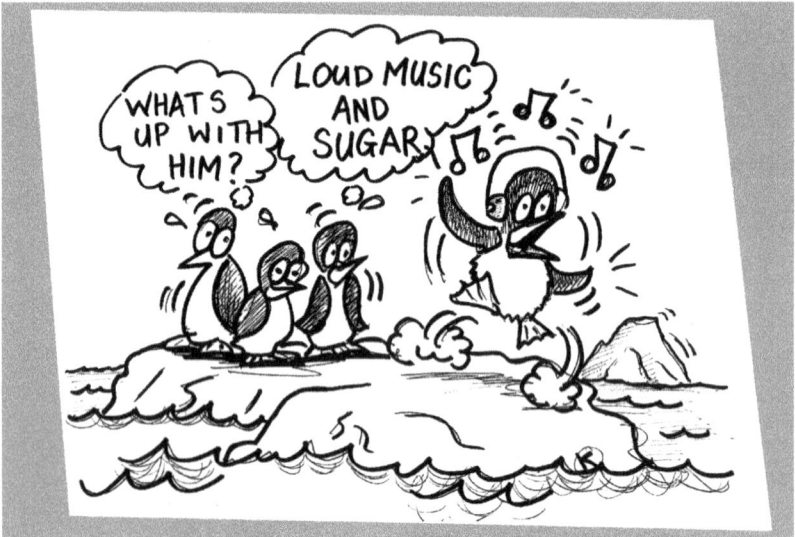

So beware and be aware of sugar. Powering your brain requires just the right amount of fuel – not too much, not too little – a high sugar diet may lead your body to a state where it can no longer keep the correct balance of glucose and insulin. Once you're there you're heading towards diabetes, you may already be obese, and your life line may be shrinking.

Fat and your brain

When I was at school my PE teacher always called us 'fatheads' as he rapped a large bunch of keys against our skulls. That was a long time ago, but I wonder if he knew then how right he was. If you take out the water, what's left of our brain is about 60% fat, so having a fatty brain is a good thing.

But there are nice fats and there are the downright bad fats. Many foods, including most of the fast food you eat, have been cooked in oil that is not one of the good fats. While the occasional snack may do you no apparent harm, eating the bad fats all the time is like using cheap oil in a formula one racing car – eventually you will have problems. Here's some of the science to explain why.

FUN FACT:
SCURVY, FROM A LACK
OF VITAMIN C, KILLED
MORE SAILORS IN THE
"AGE OF SAIL" THAN
THE WHOLE AMERICAN
CIVIL WAR.

The fats we must eat to build our brains are called essential fatty acids (EFAs). There are two kinds – omega-3 and omega-6. The brain has the highest content of omega-3 fatty acids found in the body. You find them in the outer coating of the neurons where the neurotransmitters bind to allow the cell to communicate, and in the myelin, which insulates the neurons. EFAs are long chain molecules that are woven into the fabric of the cell membranes and they provide flexibility. If the brain cell membranes become too stiff, key brain chemicals can't do their jobs, and brain activities such as learning, reaction speeds and memory start to decline.

Other fats you may eat (think French fries) are also long chain molecules, but they lack the flexibility of the omega fats. As they

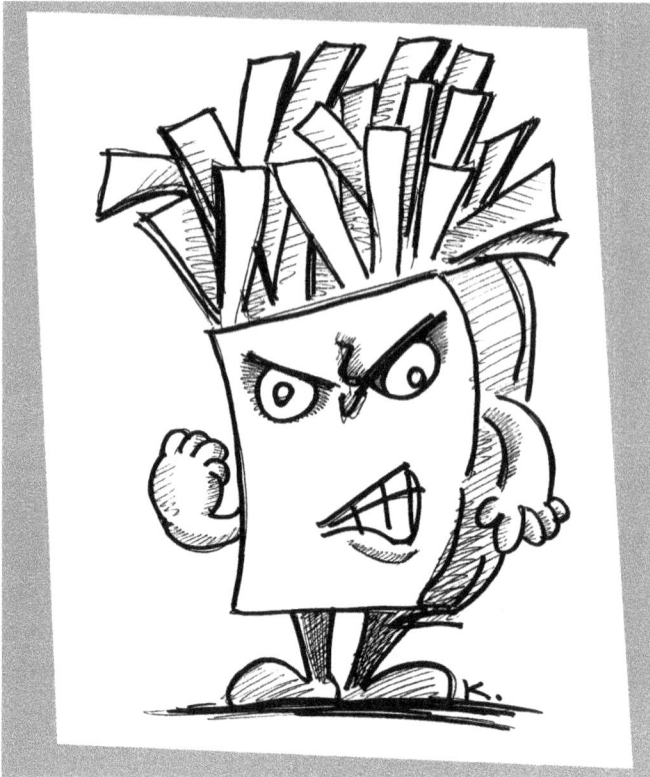

replace the omega-3 in the cell membranes, the cells become more rigid and their function is impaired. It's as simple as that.

Some of the bad fats you may have heard of are 'trans-fats', or the *trans fatty acids*. You can get these from fatty meat, and they are also created chemically during cooking with vegetable oil. They are not 'essential' fats but there are plenty in oil-fried food. They are the reasons that people who wish to remain as healthy as possible generally avoid fast food restaurants and deep fried foods.

As you know, neurons only have to do one thing – communicate by sending an electro-chemical message down their myelin fat coated axons. The raw materials for making myelin are the EFAs. The best source of them is seafood, particularly oily fish from cold water sources, and some plants, like chia seeds and walnuts. Some people take fish or krill oil nutritional supplements that have brain benefits if they don't eat sufficient EFAs in their diet.

Jean Carper, author of *Your Miracle Brain*, states that the type of fat you put into your body might be the most important decision you make on behalf of your brain throughout your lifetime. And it is not only our mental capacities that depend on the right proportion of fats, but also our longevity and vulnerability to depression. Research shows that animals fed the wrong fats end up dumber than animals fed the right fats. In fact one of the best ways to screw up the perfectly good brain you are born with is to eat the wrong fats – at any age.

If you have ever seen butter go bad you know what going 'rancid' means. It's a term that describes the oxidation of the fat. It can happen in the brain fat too. Once it has been oxidised – chemically altered after a reaction with oxygen – fats are pretty much useless to us and some of the by-products, called 'free radicals', are toxic.

You may have heard of 'antioxidants', which we can also include in our diet. The fats in our brain are pretty sensitive to oxidation but if we eat an array of antioxidants we can maintain them and keep our brains healthy. One of the advantages of modern life is the availability of these antioxidants – you get them in fruits, vegetables and spices. Avocados are good, also berries (especially blueberries), coffee and freshly brewed leaf tea (not the bottled kind). Eggs, nuts and seeds are good sources of brain nutrients too. Dark green vegetables, like spinach, are packed full of antioxidants. Neurosurgeon Dr Larry McCleary says they have the antioxidant power to 'whip oxygen free radicals like Popeye whipped Bluto.' McCleary says eating dark green vegetables will slow brain aging, improve memory, and enhance dexterity.

Brain cells are the most sensitive cells in your body to many of the nutrients and dietary chemicals you eat in your diet. To maximise the efficiency of your brain you need the best diet available. If you get it right by ensuring your lifestyle includes both mental stimulation and physical exercise, you can have a dramatic impact on how well your brain works and your longevity.

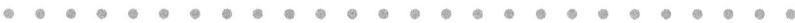

THINK ABOUT IT

* Look up www.glycemicindex.com and work out the Glycemic Index of the foods you eat regularly.
* Are they fast burning high GI, or slow-burning low GI foods?

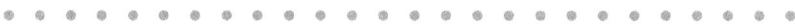

A MESSAGE TO YOUR TEACHERS

Are you happy with your school canteen and what it serves the kids? Throughout my teaching career there appeared every year or so some groovy young hip teacher, usually vegetarian, who, at staff meetings railed against the foods in the canteen and sometimes got enough support to push through some changes in what was offered. Know the type? Then, slowly, the foods reverted to what they were before: the lowest common denominator – what's easiest to prepare, makes profit, or what the kids demand, irrespective of their health.

Few of your students will get scurvy or kwashiorkor eating at the school canteen, but you know what? Those young teachers are 100% right. School canteens need to model good diets. You are setting the standards people could follow their entire lives. And, once more, as diet can directly affect behaviour, it's just possible that your classes will be easier to teach, the students will achieve greater things, and teaching will be like it's supposed to be – a joy.

A MESSAGE TO YOUR PARENTS

Parenting is a relentless task. The media continually blasts out messages as to why you're supposed to be eating which fast food, and you *know* what's good for you, but.... our kids can be so persuasive!

A diet of brain food – low GI fruits and vegetables, good fats and oils, sufficient proteins, minerals and vitamins, can be hard work. But good habits started in the early years may persist throughout a very long and healthy life. Isn't that what we all want for our kids?

One more thing: If you're a parent of boys I recommend you read *Boys Adrift*, by Dr Leonard Sax. There is an epidemic of low motivation among Western male youth, and one of the factors he presents strong evidence for is diet related. Not what you may think either. We may be eating dangerous amounts of chemicals called *phthalates* and *bisphenol A* that we ingest with our food because they have been wrapped or cooked in plastics. These chemicals give water that 'plasticky' taste you sometimes get in water bottles, and they leach out of the plastics we use all the time with our food. They affect kids because they act like female hormones. Sax calls them 'endocrine disruptors' and he suggests they are contributing to girls reaching puberty earlier (now as young as eight!) and boys later (perhaps 14 or 15) and they're also linked to shrunken motivation centres in boys' brains.

Sax's strong advice includes: avoid reheating foods in the microwave in plastic containers or wraps (use glass instead), and avoid plastic drink bottles, dummies, chewable PVC baby toys etc.

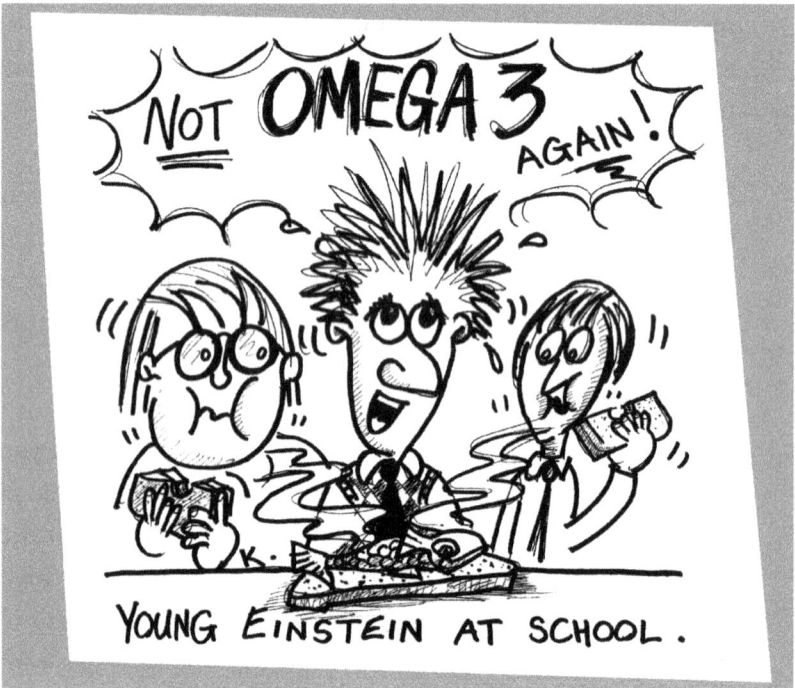

YOUNG EINSTEIN AT SCHOOL.

Section 3.

How Now to Your Future?

Now you understand a bit about the structure and function of your brain and how to get it running smoothly and efficiently, here's a little more about the biochemistry of your brain and how it's changing in your teenage years. The continual pruning and growth of your neurons is helping you prepare for adulthood and all the challenges and responsibilities that are ahead.

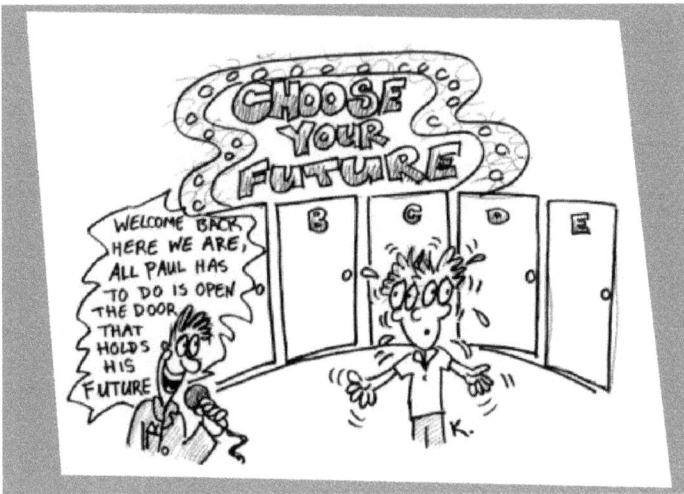

This section takes you through some of the confusing changes you'll be noticing and the reasons why you are starting to do things which a few years ago would never have crossed your mind. The teen years may present risks to you and stresses you have never dreamed of before, but it will also present you with opportunities which you can choose to accept, or not. These years are all about you! This is when you forge much of the identity you take into the rest of your life. Learning and building upon your strengths and finding strategies with which to develop your weaknesses will help immeasurably.

In these years you are preparing yourself for independence and adulthood. But you are still a 'learning sponge' so it's a great time for school, even if there are challenges to face and conquer along the way. What you have in your head, as Anne Gosline put it in *New Scientist*, is the potential to "sculpt your brain into lean, mean processing machines." Now is the time, make the most of it.

Chapter 8

Something is Happening to Your Brain!

. . . .

IN THIS CHAPTER YOU WILL LEARN

✦ How your brain is changing during the important teenage years.
✦ Why these changes are necessary.

. . . .

You are 'adolescent'!

What's the big deal? Well, for some cultures and language groups across the world it's not a big deal at all. Some don't even have a word for adolescence, and they appear to have seamless transitions from childhood to adulthood. Psychologist, Dr Robert Epstein, found more than a hundred cultures like this, and argues that in western societies kids are being 'infantilised' in a way that never happened in the pre-industrial age. Our great grandparents may have become apprentices and begun a working life at thirteen. They 'grew up fast' with no time for an extended childhood, so they missed the challenges and problems we've come to expect in the teen years. If you are thirteen do you feel ready for a nine hour workday, every day?

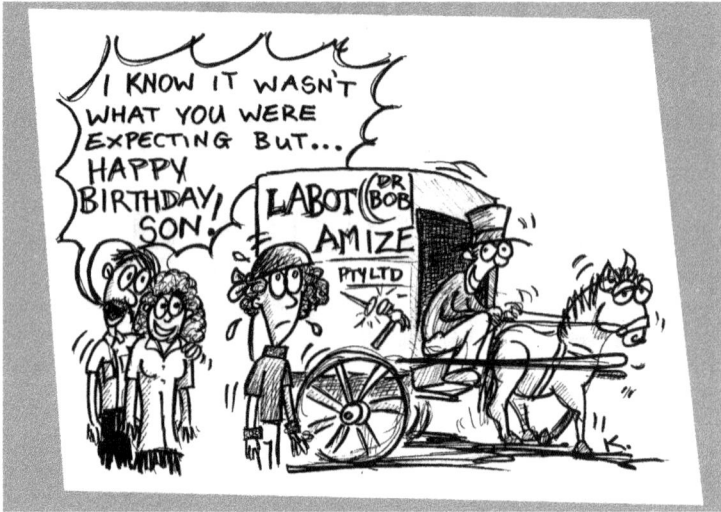

The evidence that adolescence is longer now than ever before is strong. Sometimes it lasts up to 15 years, when it used to be just three or four years. Puberty now regularly occurs earlier these days, especially for girls, than it did even 50 years ago, and as psychologist Dr Dan Willingham says, puberty is the beginning of adolescence, and these days, with school, college, then university going on and on (and on and on!) some might not become 'adult' until after these activities are all over – sometimes by the age of 25!

So what are most neuroscientists and educators saying about you? Well, we know the changes probably all started when you were between eight and ten years of age. This is the end of the *critical period* when your brain changed from a learning sponge to something you're going to have to work to use properly in the future. Have you ever wondered how you ever learned to speak without studying? Perhaps you learned two or three languages when still a toddler. You learned your language when your brain was in a critical period. Those years are gone for teenagers and that means you may have to work harder for the same result. However, you're still in a prime learning age and your brain is a powerful instrument. The teenage years are extraordinary learning times you can choose to make the most of.

One of the tasks you can set for yourself in your teens is to find out your personal learning style and how best you learn. Knowing these will help make learning difficult things more efficient and therefore easier. All you need is the confidence and the motivation and you can learn and do amazing things.

When you were about ten years old your brain had many billions more synapses than you'll need when you're an adult. It started a period of active 'synaptic pruning' (remember: synapses are the connections between neurons.) Between the age of ten and thirteen you could be losing as many as 30,000 synapses *every*

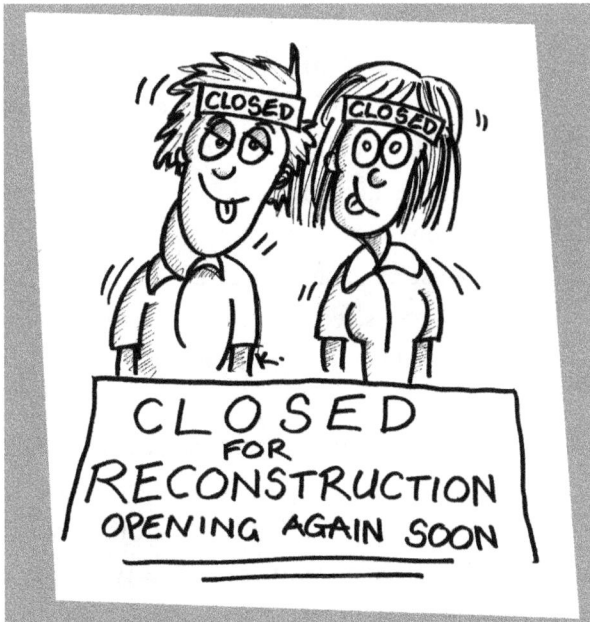

second. What your brain is doing is getting rid of the weakest connections and keeping those that are useful. It's a ruthless process that could clear away about half of them. Your brain is specializing itself based on its experience to date and, according to Dr Epstein, your memory and intelligence actually peaks in these years.

FUN FACT:
THE BRAIN REACHES
FULL MATURITY WHEN
IT IS ABOUT 25
YEARS OLD.

This pruning is essential for another reason. The axons of the neurones you will keep are going through continued myelinisation (myelin coating) to make them work faster and more efficiently.

Your brain's frontal lobes are being renovated during this stage. These lobes are the areas which make you a civilized human being. They control planning, judgment, wisdom, kindness, and consideration. Psychologist, Andrew Fuller, says someone should hang a sign on teenagers' frontal lobes saying 'CLOSED FOR RECONSTRUCTION'. This is a bit misleading – of course you are already 'civilised' and you make decisions and judgements every day. It's just that perhaps they'll be different decisions in five or ten years time as your judgement matures. And don't worry; all this makes perfect sense to evolutionary biologists who say it only happens because it's been selected for over millions of years, and that it must be an advantage to us as a species.

For the early teen years, your brain seems to be ruled by parts other than the frontal lobes. Your amygdala has a great time – making you more emotional, ready for a fight or running away ('fight or flight'), and more inclined towards romance (you start showing sexual interest in other people). The trouble is your ability to forward plan and control your impulses may seem switched off, so in most cultures your parents are meant to plan for you. That's their job and it's important – too much freedom now can be a disaster for you, so give them a break sometimes, *please*.

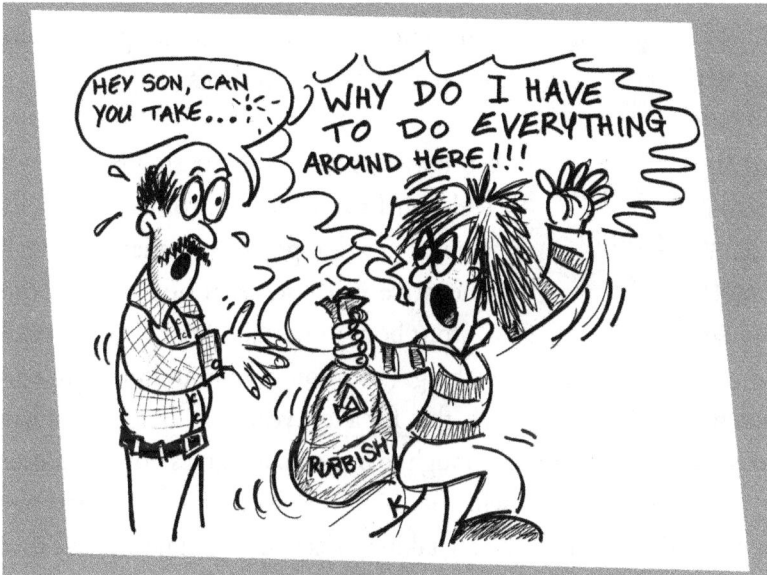

At twelve or thirteen you're really about to grow. In the next few years you may put on 20 kilograms and grow 50 centimetres taller; you may get pimples and hairy and see other obvious changes taking place. Your friends may become especially important now. Popularity for some people is more necessary than ever – some kids will take big risks to gain peer acceptance. You will probably spend a lot more time talking with your peers than to adults. You may sometimes go 'ballistic' when asked to take out the trash, and wonder why you have to do *everything*. You will be developing your sexual identity and your need for privacy may grow considerably. I bet you already have a 'KEEP OUT' sign on your bedroom door.

As you live through your teens and start part time work, or apprenticeships, you may prove to be a phenomenally reliable employee and an excellent driver (it's the 21-25 year olds who have more accidents, so be warned) and you may be goal orientated, knowing exactly what you want to do and how to get there. On the other hand, perhaps you don't have a clue, and that's okay too.

FUN FACT:
A 12 YEAR OLD'S
BRAIN MAY BE
PRUNING AS MANY
AS 30,000 SYNAPSES
EVER SECOND!

You may also be feeling stressed because you feel you have little control over your life. Things may happen to you that seem really negative in these years but later on they won't be as important. Your views on many things (sex, money, your future) might be so different from your family's, that for a few years you are going to have conflict. This is common enough to be normal, but it's not compulsory, so don't wish it on yourself. You might also be feeling confused, angry or aggressive. You're probably taking risks you would never have done a few years ago. You may be experimenting with drugs or alcohol. You may be breaking your parents' hearts but think that's not your problem! Or you may be a sweet teen sailing through without any of these issues.

All of us find our own pathway, and most of us survive well. You've just got to make sure that you're one of the survivors.

THINK ABOUT IT

* Where are you on these 'normal' scales?
* Mark where you think you are now and check back in a year or two to see if you have changed.

1   2   3   4   5   6   7   8   9   10
Stressed .... Relaxed.

1   2   3   4   5   6   7   8   9   10
Irresponsible .... Responsible.

1   2   3   4   5   6   7   8   9   10
Inconsistent .... Totally reliable.

Name: _____ Date _____

A MESSAGE TO YOUR TEACHERS

Isn't middle school fun? Primary school teachers look at middle schools with fear and trepidation – how do middle school teachers survive? The kids can seem unruly, ill-mannered and ill-disciplined as they navigate through adolescence towards adulthood. The teachers can appear frazzled and worn out by an endless supply of teenagers moving through the school. But middle school is where the

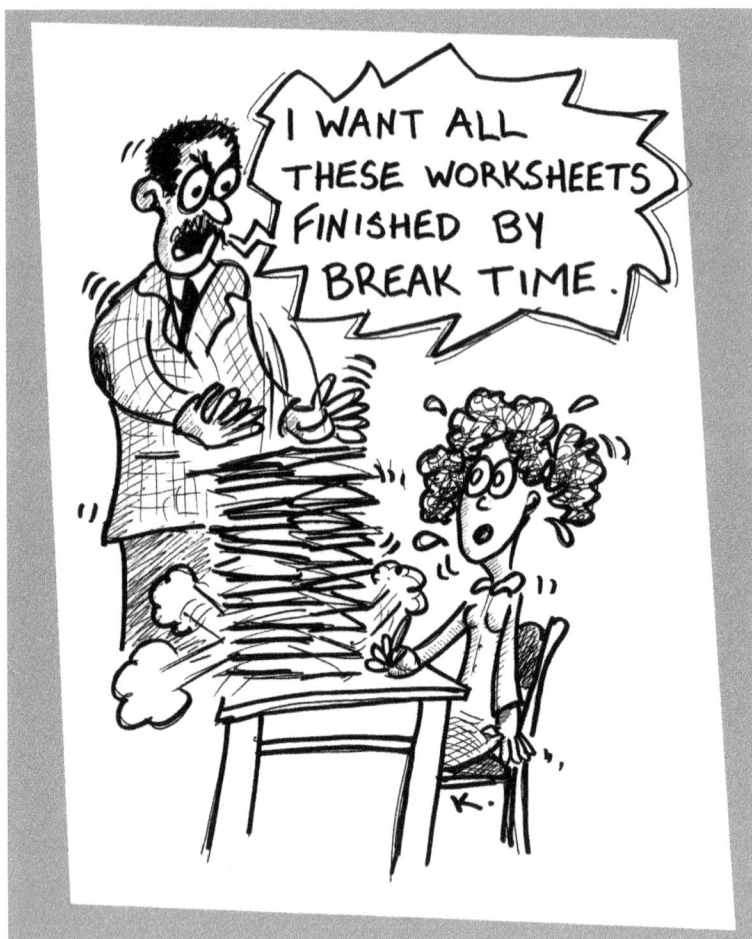

action is. It's where personalities really develop and kids get a skill base that will set them up for the rest of their lives. And teachers can really make a difference.

Teaching nowadays is different to when I first started. I cringe at some of the learning tasks I used to set, believing I was teaching. For example, I'd sometimes set worksheets for homework that were nothing more than 'busywork' because that's what I was told to do by the school's 'homework policy'. What a waste of good learning opportunities or family time!

With our increasing knowledge about how the brain learns, and developing brain-based learning strategies that use this knowledge, we will see dramatic changes over the next century to education. A 'one size fits all' teaching program is no longer valid. We need to be teaching the individual, not the mob, because everyone learns differently. Many teachers need to up-skill and discard those strategies that waste kids' time.

The wheels of change move slowly, and it might take a hundred years for the education culture to change, so the sooner we start the better. It's in everyone's interest to turn all our schools into places where learning is efficient and maximised. So go forth, get trained, read some books, and teach with the brain in mind.

A MESSAGE TO YOUR PARENTS

You may know your son or daughter better than anyone, and you have played, and will continue to play, a role as a highly significant adult in their lives. But your teenagers may astound you, confuse you, and stretch your relationship to its limits. Sometimes some of the things they say and do can be startling or downright hurtful. They can scream at you one minute, and then want to borrow the car the next. They can be ungrateful little brats one hour, and delightful young adults the next, all the time needing your love and support.

Teenagers have phenomenal brains and can learn incredible amounts of new material much faster than you can. They are at the peak of their learning years and whilst so much is going on in their lives and their bodies, it's no wonder that they can be hard to fathom sometimes. You may not understand the sudden mood swings or tantrums some teens have, but you need to accept them, and be patient. Your teen needs your support but will demand increasingly more independence from you. This 'letting go' can be hard for some parents but watching kids rise to meet challenging responsibilities given to them gives you pride in their abilities and opportunities to celebrate their success.

Teens need to be given responsibility. They need to be trusted, and if they make mistakes, they need to be forgiven and trusted again. Parents' input can be crucial to the success of the developing new adult. The most crucial discovery your teens are in the process of working out is their identity – who they will be as adults, how they will find their place in the world and how they can do it whilst still feeling good about themselves.

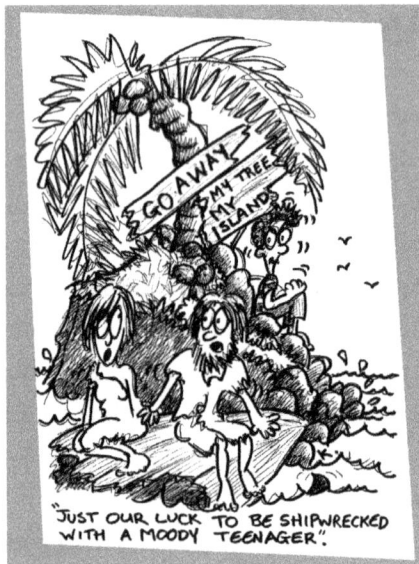

"JUST OUR LUCK TO BE SHIPWRECKED WITH A MOODY TEENAGER".

Chapter 9

Hormones

. . . .

IN THIS CHAPTER YOU WILL LEARN

+ Four major hormones that affect your brain's mood.
+ The hormones you should try and limit and those you may want more of.

. . . .

*D*o the adults around you roll their eyes at your actions, shrug their shoulders and say '*hormones!*' as if this explains everything?

Well, you now know that it is your brain, and its massive reorganisation, that's as much to blame for what's going on as anything else. But it is also worth knowing what the hormones are that people are talking about, how they affect you and what you can do about them.

In many ways teenagers are at the mercy of their hormones. So is everyone else, but in *your* body, dramatic changes are taking place in nearly every part. Hormones are chemical 'messengers' released by glands in the body to control other parts. You may have heard of some of the glands – the pituitary, the adrenal, and the pineal glands for example. The hormones they release do everything, from creating your sleep patterns, to stopping you urinating during the night (try going 9 or 10 hours during the day without a wee!). You'll be learning about two of them, testosterone and oestrogen (the sex hormones) in Chapter 12, as they will be starting to really do their thing in your conversion from child to adult during your teen years.

But what about your brain? This Chapter is mainly about the four main hormones you should know about that put you into your moods. Moods have a dramatic effect on your ability to concentrate and therefore the efficiency of your learning. All four of these hormones play multiple roles, but for now we'll focus on how they affect the way you feel, and what you can do to ensure positive moods. Two of them are nicer than the other two, but let's look at the two you may want less of in your daily life first, adrenalin and cortisol, and then look at those which you want to promote, serotonin and dopamine.

Hormones you need to limit

Adrenalin

Adrenalin gives you power. I was snorkelling with my friend Robert once, and a sea snake swam towards us. Sea snakes are masters of their environment and have little to fear from us, therefore are usually very safe to be near, even though most are extremely poisonous. Robert didn't think of that. The snake swam towards him, he kicked at it wildly, and his flippers came off. He panicked and the next thing he knew he was standing two meters out of the water, on a barnacle covered rock. He had no memory of how he got there. Adrenalin had kicked his amygdala (the part of his brain that controls the 'flight or fight' response) into taking control of his body – and up he went. This is survival at its most basic. I don't know what happened to the poor snake.

> FUN FACT:
> MUSIC TRIGGERS
> THE RELEASE OF
> DOPAMINE – THE
> SAME PLEASURE
> HORMONE YOU GET
> DURING SEX, AND
> EATING.

You may not be swimming with sea snakes, but it is possible for people to build up high levels of adrenalin in a number of ways even without scary things, and sometimes it's fun to get an 'adrenalin buzz. We get them from roller coasters and other exciting rides, or even scary movies. However, too much for too long can give you a mood you might not want.

How can you tell if you have high adrenalin? Clinical psychologist Andrew Fuller is an expert on this and the questions below come from his work (see *Tricky Kids*).

If you answer yes to a lot of these questions it is possible you have high adrenalin levels.

* Do you feel silly, or hyperactive?

* Is it hard to fall asleep?

* Do you have lots of energy?

* Do you 'spit the dummy' and run off?

* Do you argue a lot?

* Do you lose concentration?

* Are you worried about trying new things?

* Are you busy without achieving much?

If you have a high adrenalin level, how do you get it down? There are a few easy things you can do. If you can, work with your family or friends to help you calm down by having quiet times. Perhaps you could learn to meditate, or do repetitious or ritual things that are easy. Talk with an adult you trust, perhaps a parent, teacher or school counsellor. Try to be where you feel safe as much as possible. These are things *you* can control, though maybe you will need some help, so don't be afraid to ask for it.

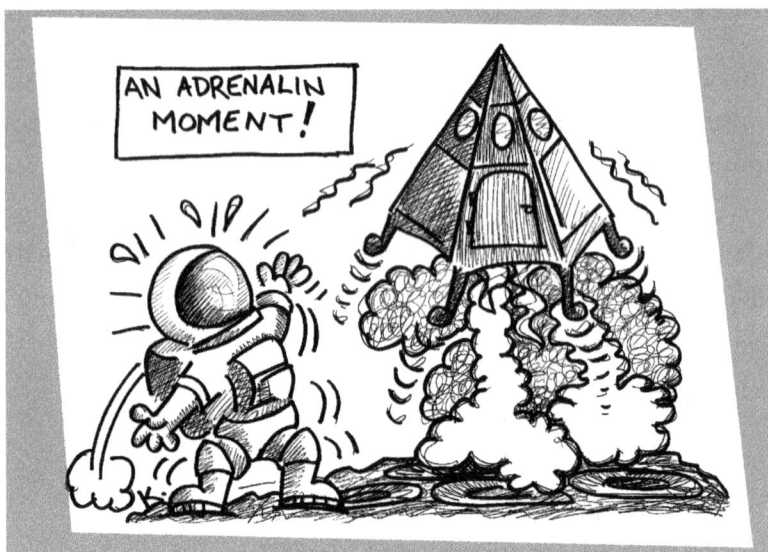

Cortisol

Cortisol is the second hormone I warned you about. Watch out for it because it is released during times of stress, and often follows adrenalin in a double whammy. I saw a two year old boy fall into a pool once and nearly drown. We rescued him and he needed resuscitating, but he didn't seem particularly phased by the experience. His mother however was hysterical. She couldn't speak, she screamed and screamed and pulled out her hair. She was a mess. Cortisol does this. In high levels, it blocks your ability to think clearly and speak your thoughts. The boy's mother had way too much cortisol (and adrenalin as well) for normal functioning, for at least a few minutes.

How can you tell if you have too much? Again, answer these questions:

* Do you find it hard to express your thoughts?

* Are you worried or on edge?

* Are you bullied regularly?

* Are you upset easily?

* Are you defensive and overreact to things?

* Do you find it difficult to prioritise?

* Do you smell more? Cortisol makes your sweat smell sour.

FUN FACT:
THE BRAIN PRODUCES
MORE THAN 50
IDENTIFIED ACTIVE
CHEMICALS WHICH ACT
LIKE DRUGS.

If you have high cortisol for a long period it will become a problem. What are you going to do? Firstly, you have to be somewhere you feel safe, away from violence or humiliation. If that's not where you spend most of the day, talk to someone – a school counsellor, parent or adult friend about how you feel. Try not to eat too much sugar, and drink lots of water (cortisol is soluble). Go to bed early and get more sleep. Don't exacerbate the situation by playing violent video games or watching violent movies. Listen to soothing music; put away your violent hip hop MP3s for a while – you know which ones I mean.

These are things *you* can control. If you need help consider phoning one of the counselling agencies listed at the back of this book.

Hormones you may want more of.

Dopamine

Dopamine is cool. It's 'the party animal of the neurochemical world'. We want dopamine because it makes us feel switched on and positive.

Many neuroscientists think that dopamine might be the one neurotransmitter that is the bottom line for pleasure. Dopamine binds to the pleasure centres of the brain. Without it you experience little pleasure.

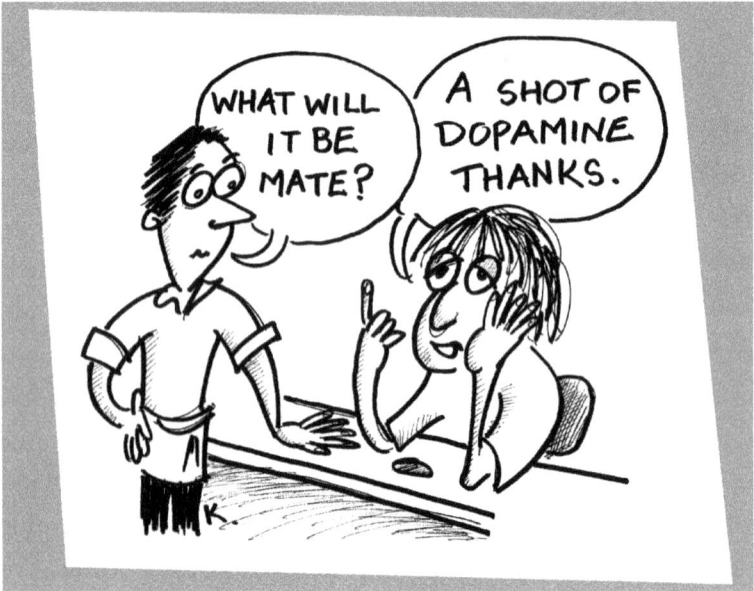

Eight or nine year old kids have an adult dose. But teenagers sometimes get ripped off. Your dopamine levels may have dropped over the last few years. How can you tell if you're low on dopamine? Answer these questions (based on Fuller 2007):

✳ Do you have trouble focusing or concentrating?

✳ Are you hard to motivate?

✳ When you finish something do you lack pride in what you have done?

✳ Are you lethargic and tired all the time?

✳ Is everything boring?

Too many yeses here, and you may need more dopamine. Where do you get it? Easy – your brain will make it for you if you exercise it in the right way. Try repetitive sports like swimming, or ping pong, or challenging games and solving problems. Spend more time with your friends and family and be more social. Try new things, seek success. Do things that make you laugh, especially with other people but you can also laugh anytime – even a fake laugh has benefit. You can eat better too – include omega 3 and 6 in your diet (see Chapter 7).

These are things *you* can control.

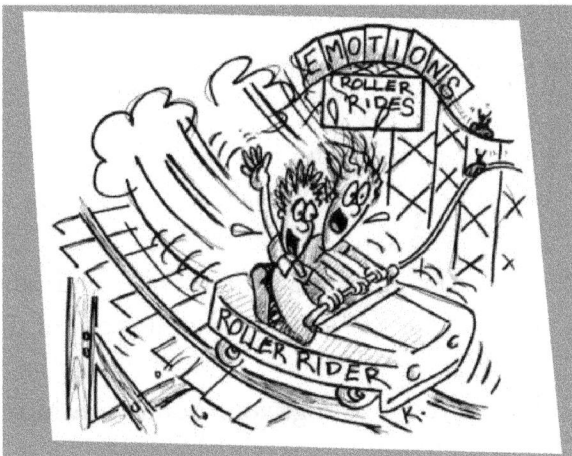

Serotonin

Serotonin is another beauty – the feel good hormone of choice, because it acts by calming you rather than revving you up like dopamine. If you miss out on this one it is a depressing experience, as lack of it is linked to depression. Fuller calls it the 'quiet achiever', giving you a slow high that makes you feel good and calm, and in control.

How can you tell if you don't have enough serotonin? Answer these questions:

* Are you sullen and uncommunicative?

* Is it hard to get out of bed in the morning?

* Are you hard to please, nothing ever good enough?

* Is everything just too hard?

* Are you sad or depressed?

* Do you avoid looking others in the eye? (eg your parents, teachers, friends?)

* Do you try to avoid your family's activities?

The good news is that serotonin is easy to make. You get it from exercise – even just walking. You get it by spending time with friends or family who support you and make you feel like you belong. You get it by accepting responsibility and taking some control. You get it from cuddling. In fact, it is one of the reasons massage is popular, as serotonin is raised during any positive contact. If you have a pet dog, your bond with him or her is probably serotonin based.

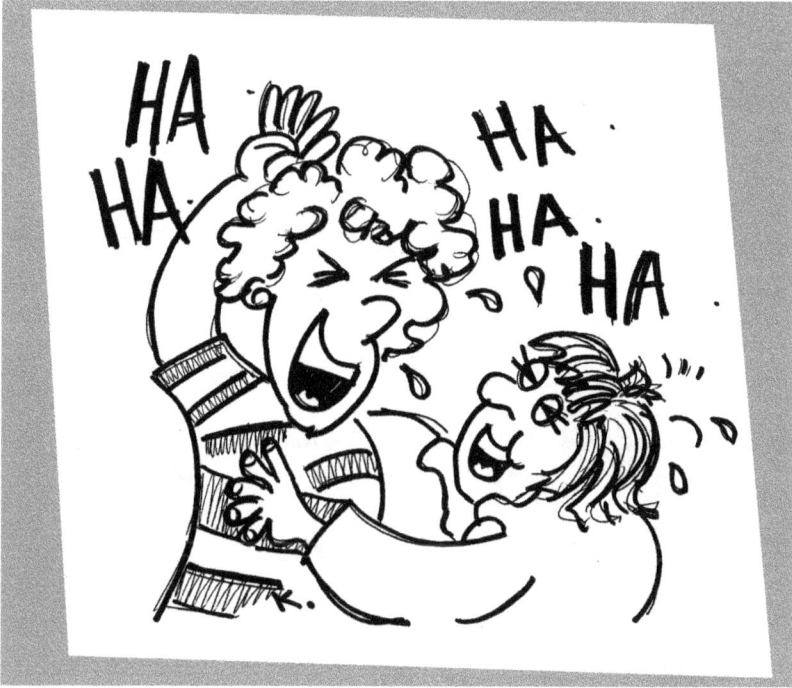

A MESSAGE TO YOUR TEACHERS

Middle school teachers have the best of both worlds. They see children arrive at their schools and young adults leave, proud and learned, ready for the next challenge. That's the theory anyway. In reality you have classes full of kids all at different stages of puberty. They often come from different backgrounds and have wide ranging levels of confidence and motivation and it's your job to teach each of them a million things.

Dopamine and serotonin are the hormones teachers need to promote in school. The right amount of these and learning is a breeze. Teachers who can incorporate laughter and enjoyment in their lessons teach more.

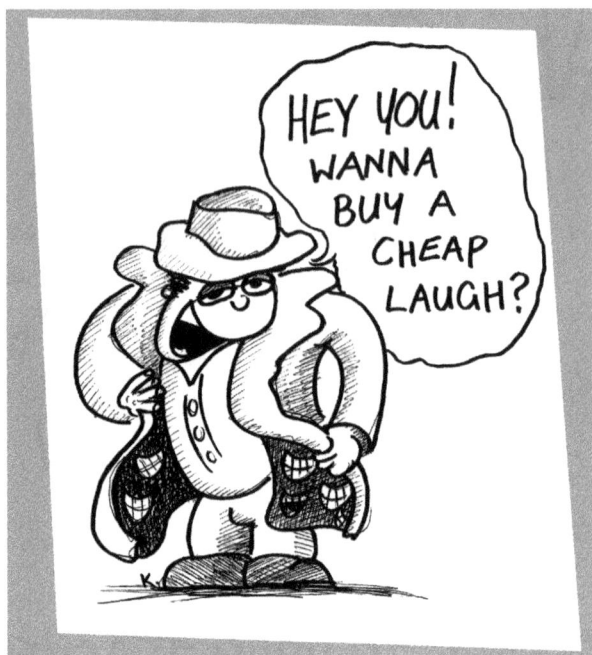

There is room, of course, for the stress hormones. A little stress can ensure peak performance and give students the edge. It wakes them up and can help focus attention. Too much stress, however, kills learning. Angry or terrified students have great difficulty in learning school programs. Did you learn about Maslow's 'hierarchy of needs' at teachers college? The basic needs of food, water, shelter, toilets, friendships and safety must be met before anyone can develop their self esteem and reach the 'self actualisation' stage.

A lack of safety for a student will build up cortisol levels and stressed students often perform badly. If they are being bullied or harassed at school by students or teachers, or are living a nightmare at home, the lack of a feeling of safety will heavily impact their self esteem and hence their level of learning.

In-school stressors can also so consume a student before an event that they are completely distracted from anything else (making a student speak publicly can a big one). Good teaching takes this into account and allows students to improve their skills in all areas when they are ready. As they build their confidence, through mastering the small steps along the way, stress is relieved.

A MESSAGE TO YOUR PARENTS

Be aware that your teenage children still need guidance. If they become isolated from you, or you continue to treat them like children, then they may get trapped in what has become known as 'teen culture' – continuing and building upon something which didn't exist a few years ago. If they are learning everything they know from their peers, without guidance from you, then it's no wonder they get confused – their friends are confused too!

Teenagers treated like adults tend to respond like adults. Here's a little secret: teenagers are not *especially* affected by hormones, I mean, any more than we are – we all have them and they work in the same way. So whilst there is truth in what I said above that suits teens, it also suits most of us. The kids are just learning to cope and build their independence in this world, as we did. We are all ruled by our biology.

Give your kids a break. Treat them with the respect they deserve. Allow them to make mistakes they will learn from. It's your job to ensure they only make small mistakes they can bounce back from, not the disastrous kind. Remember the thrill about how great it was to be a parent when they were born? Nothing has changed – it's still the best thing in the world.

Chapter 10

A Risky Future

IN THIS CHAPTER YOU WILL LEARN

* Why risk taking can be fun, and necessary.
* About some of the major risks you may face and why.

Taking Risks

Taking risks is a big thing for many teenagers. Some kids like to take risks for reasons that can best be explained by *'because I felt like it!!!'* Some kids don't think they take risks at all, though of course we all must, to stay alive (you take a risk every time you go in a car, cross the road, eat take-away foods). Risks can just be about trying out something new – like a new game, meeting new people, learning to drive. If you don't take risks you do nothing – which is a risk in itself.

Are you a big risk taker? First in line at the roller coaster? Climbed any flagpoles lately? Do you skate, surf, race shopping carts, ride motorbikes, play football, shoplift, argue with bullies, stare down your teachers, take drugs, get drunk? If you take risks, like roller coaster rides, that your parents are no longer interested in you'll know you have a teenage brain and they don't. Roller coasters don't mean as much to older people – and guess what, you won't understand that for ten or twenty years.

Some risk taking is so dangerous your very survival is at stake. Let me tell you a story about two brothers I used to teach. I'll rename them, Bob and John. They were cool kids, in a country town, with a single highway heading north and south. John was about 15 years old, and someone encouraged him to go car surfing. Standing on the hood of a mate's car at 80 km per hour can be fun, until you fall off, and yes, he did indeed fall. And killed himself. He was a popular kid in a small town. His funeral was a very sad affair, attended by most of the community. His brother Bob was very upset, of course. So upset, in fact, that a few days later, he honoured John's memory by taking the same risk. He went car surfing along the same stretch of road and he too fell off, within 200 meters of where his brother died. And Bob died too. One family, two brothers, two funerals, in one week! Can you imagine that?

FUN FACT: IT TAKES ABOUT SIX MINUTES FOR THE BRAIN TO BE AFFECTED BY ALCOHOL.

Some risks aren't as fatal as car surfing, but instead have a danger that is more 'perceived' than real. Roller coasters, and other fairground rides, are like this. The riders scream with fear and excitement for a few minutes and come off with shaky knees babbling '*really scary like, fantastic, let's do it again?*'

The feelings on the ride are probably the same feelings Bob and John experienced before their accidents, but kids going on these rides face no real danger of dying. Their brains just trick them into perceiving a danger that is not really there.

As a teenager I used to seek out the rides. I was also into rock climbing, caving, bush walking, horse riding, scuba diving and even sky diving. I spent three months backpacking alone in

Europe when I was 17. At 18 I used to drive too fast, and play pranks on mates. I kept funnel web spiders in my bedroom as pets. I regularly went out bush to catch poisonous snakes, and one of my first jobs was catching them in swamps swarming with crocodiles, for a university study. All these activities are risky. Some are dangerous, like horse riding. And some are just downright stupid, like speeding cars and swimming with crocodiles. Some kids I knew didn't survive these kinds of high risk activities and sometimes I can't believe how stupid I was.

But I was lucky. The worst I experienced was crashing a motorbike at 130 km/hr; spending five days in hospital and having to pay for the bike. My nickname was *Reckless Derek*! But rock climbing, as long as you're using ropes correctly, is not so bad. And most of the time, I never really felt under threat when engaged in these risky sports. I trusted the equipment and my own inflated view of my abilities. Oh, except for sky diving. I only ever did two jumps, but both times had malfunctions with my parachute, so I concluded that perhaps this was not really my sport (although I told my mates I quit because it was too expensive to continue).

I sometimes think I must have been a late developer – my frontal cortex doesn't seem to have taken control until I was about 25, which was about the time I said no to bungee jumping and people stopped calling me *Reckless Derek* (really – I even published using this nickname!)

Insurance companies know all about these risk taking years, and it's no coincidence that the premiums are often higher for the under twenty fives.

Why do people take risks?

You already know. It's your developing frontal cortex that likes to ignore risk, and that lovely dopamine, your party hormone, which makes you feel great. Dopamine is the hormone that is linked to the pleasure centres of the brain. You wouldn't know you were having pleasure without it. You already know that when a neuron fires its little electric pulses down its axon to the synaptic cleft between it and the next neuron in the chain, the message gets sent across the gap by chemicals called neurotransmitters. Dopamine is the neurotransmitter that screams out 'yippee!' It passes the message on that you are thrilled or excited and this feels good. So you're likely to want more.

The more the dopamine system is activated the more pleasure you feel. If you like pleasure, you'll look for something that gives you high levels of dopamine. Excitement can be addictive. Some people need it more and more and do wilder and wilder things, taking major risks, to get it. All brains are unique and some people may have to try riskier activities (like BASE jumping for instance) to get the same feelings of pleasure in their brains as others who do less risky things.

Neuroscientists and educators know that an adolescent's brain is different to that same brain in both childhood and adulthood. But why? There is some evidence that teenagers' dopamine levels drop after they leave childhood. This can leave your brain craving a dopamine 'hit'. Situations that used to give you enough dopamine when you were younger no longer work as well. Excitement can be different for you now, because, as we have seen, your frontal lobes are under reconstruction. They are not yet ready to help you, their owner, make reasoned judgements or long term logical plans. So the possible consequences of risky activities may not even be apparent. Or if they are, it may just add to the excitement.

Adolescence can be a really confusing time, and the mixed messages coming from adults are a major problem. Think of sex, drugs, and rock and roll. Look around you. It's hard not to conclude from TV and billboards, music, magazines and books that humans are sex obsessed, but you're told not to *do it*. Adults tell you to say 'no' to drugs, while they drink alcohol and smoke tobacco with abandon. Most of the rock and roll messages that come to you are written by adults, while other adults say, 'oh no, you shouldn't behave like *that!*'

What's a teenager supposed to make of mixed messages like this? To help let's look at some of the major risks you might be tempted by.

Major risks for teenagers

There are, of course, millions of risks, but here are a few that especially affect teenagers.

* Illegal Drugs

* Alcohol

* Sex

* Eating Junk

* Wild Behaviour

* Video Games

* Bullying/Cyberbullying

* Your behaviour and your parents

Illegal drugs

Why do people risk death and destruction, their health and their wealth, by taking drugs for pleasure? The answer is dopamine. Yes, the same substance you already make in normal day to day operation.

Without going into the fine details, here's a general idea of how many of the different illegal drugs work:

Dopamine, as you already know, is a neurotransmitter (among other things) that is released by one axon to excite the dendrites of the next neuron. Once it's done its job, it shifts back across the synapse and is stored again in the first axon for the next zap of electricity to set it free. Many drugs that give you pleasure work by blocking this re-uptake of dopamine so that it remains in the synapse. Dopamine then builds up and you continue to feel pleasure, and even greater feelings of pleasure, as the concentration gets higher. You are 'high' because your dopamine levels are high.

There are two things you need to know well about these drugs. The first thing is that you are at a higher risk of becoming an addict when you are a teenager than any other time of your life. Sorry, it's just something about your brains. If you start using drugs (and this goes for tobacco and alcohol too) before you are 15, then you are four times more likely to become an addict than a 21 year old.

The second thing you need to know is that, whilst you are a teenager and your brain is reconstructing and pruning and learning and everything else it needs to do, it is more easily damaged – permanently. Damage means loss of memory, inability to think clearly, perhaps schizophrenia, depression, suicidal thoughts and so on. This isn't rocket science. If there's ever a time that you shouldn't mess around with your brain and use these drugs, it's during adolescence. I am going to repeat this message: Adolescence is a *REALLY* bad time to use these drugs. Any other time is just really bad! So I'll repeat it again:

Warning: A teenager's brain is vastly more sensitive to cigarettes, alcohol and drugs than at any other time of life, so teenagers more easily become addicts.

Alcohol

Alcohol is a juggernaut of our society and, rightly or wrongly, is extremely important throughout many people's lives. Many adults, and many teenagers, drink alcohol and it never becomes an issue. But if you are regularly drinking, binge drinking, getting drunk, or are planning to, then a little information might help you in your decisions, because you are or will be, for sure, damaging your brain.

Alcohol affects the brain in direct proportion to how much you consume. You may have difficulty walking, suffer blurred vision, slurred speech, have slower reaction times, and memory problems. If you drink heavily over a long period of time you can develop problems that last even when you are sober.

You are affected by alcohol more than adults. Girls are affected more than boys. You need half the volume of alcohol adults do to become brain damaged. Brain damage first shows up as memory loss. In one study, Teenage drinkers, with an average of only two drinks a day, showed a worse memory than chronic adult alcoholics. They will not be able to repair this brain damage, ever. You are 10 times more likely to have a serious fight if you drink. You are 12 times more likely to be injured in an accident. Half of accidental deaths in teenagers involve alcohol.

So, given all this, why would you drink? Apart from fitting in with your mates and other social reasons, the reason is dopamine again. Your brain's dopamine levels rise, you feel pleasure, and as you seek more pleasure, you take more risks! This is a risk you need to make a conscious decision about. Is it worth it?

Sex

This is the section that I know you will read. As they say *"sex sells,"* so I am tempted to rewrite the entire book under this heading to make sure you get all the messages! But I guess you'd twig to that.

Everything in our community from TV and YouTube music clips and movies to advertising billboards, magazines and novels, and even your friends, seem to be saying 'Do it, do it'. But take heart. 'Doing it' is not compulsory and one of the things you can conclude from a number of large surveys about sex and teenagers is that *most teenagers don't*. Surprised? How many seventeen-year-olds are happy to admit they are still a virgin to their friends? Some do, and vow to save that special day for a special partner. Others lie. You have a teenage brain if you deny being a virgin to your friends because virginity is not cool, even though most teenagers are virgins (between 70% and 80% of teenagers remain virgins throughout their teens).

Having said that, let's look at the risks of teenage sex. The obvious one is pregnancy. This can alter your life plans dramatically, or if you don't already have a plan, may set one in stone for you. Are you ready to be a father or a mother?

Do you drink alcohol? A third of unwanted pregnancies occur when a teenage girl has sex when drunk. Couples are six times more likely to forget to use contraception when drunk than when sober. If you are sexually active, make sure you understand contraception and use it. And note, no matter what *anyone* says: the 'withdrawal method' does *not* work.

The next risk is disease. This includes HIV/AIDS, Chlamydia, herpes, hepatitis C, genital warts and syphilis. Some will kill you, others are a nuisance. But note this: about half of new HIV/AIDS victims each year are young people. And, although this disease is not the death sentence it once was, get it and you'll have to rewrite your life plan nevertheless.

FUN FACT.
THE YOUNGER A
PERSON IS TO
START USING DRUGS,
THE MORE LIKELY
HE OR SHE IS TO
BECOME ADDICTED.

Some people will still have unprotected sex despite these risks. Your job is to minimise the risks: know your partner, take precautions, and take your time. Save yourself.

And can you guess the science behind why people like to have sex? Sex increases dopamine and serotonin levels. It's something you look for to experience pleasure.

Eating junk

You learned about junk foods in Chapter 7. Just remember your brain can lie to you. *'Go on, French fries for the tenth time this week are not going to hurt, eat them, it'll be ok'.*

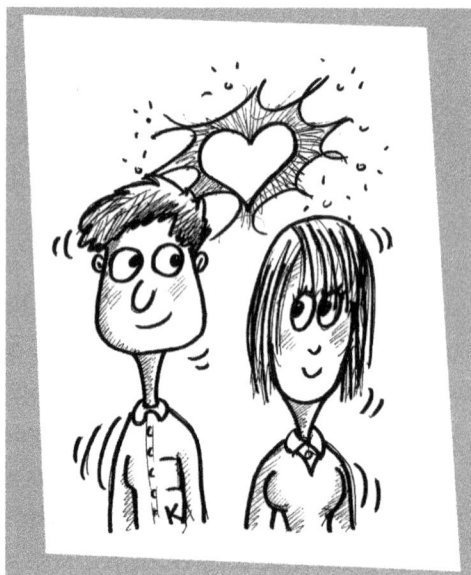

Everyone knows that the foods you like, and the foods you know are good for you, aren't necessarily the same thing. Your brain can justify anything if the desire is there. Why? Because, you guessed it, your brain craves dopamine, and eating raises dopamine levels to give you feelings of pleasure.

The risks in your diet choices may not be clear to you at first because few results are immediate. Some people make choices that lead to obesity, and then perhaps diabetes, but this takes years. These same food choices can also lead to heart disease and an early death in your forties, fifties or sixties. These seem a long way away when you're a teenager, so who cares? Well, you had better care – thirty years is not long when you look from where I am standing on the other side of fifty.

Disorders such as bulimia (binge eating, then making yourself vomit) and anorexia nervosa (eating too little food through a

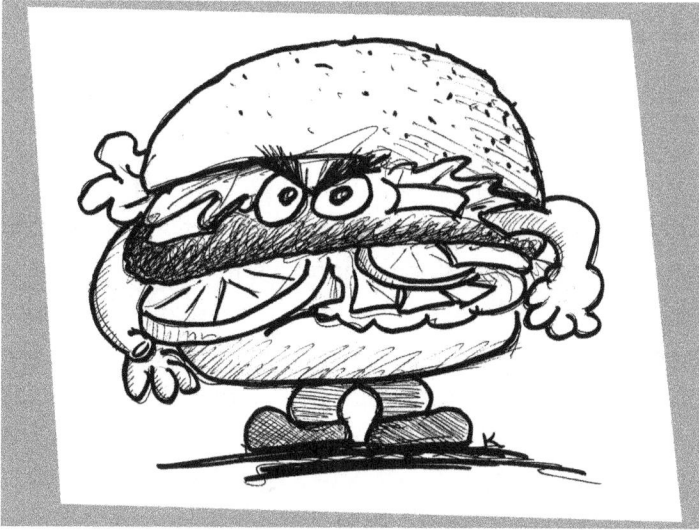

fear of putting on weight) are real psychological disorders. These problems are caused by your brain telling you lies. If you think you suffer one or other then you need to seek help. Talk to someone you trust.

Wild behaviour

You might feel the need to take part in activities that in a few years might turn your hair grey! Teenagers are notorious for driving too fast, jumping off bridges into flooded rivers, and doing other daft things. I was like that, and needed to be lucky to survive. I was 20 years old when I had a motorbike accident. I hit a ditch at 130 km/h, and the bike and I parted company. I spent my 21st birthday with my foot in a cast. I was lucky – I left the bike and flew parallel to a barbed wire fence. If I'd hit it, I would have been strips of meat drying on the wire. Lots of young people don't get lucky – read the newspapers and see how many end their lives early, or end up in a wheelchair through accidents. I had a second chance and am still here. Death was only an inch away.

You have a teenage brain if you think 'it won't happen to me!' and nothing I say here will make much of a difference to you, unless you make a conscious decision to plan to survive. Your job between now and when you turn 25 is to survive without harming yourself or others, but still have a good, productive time. Remember, most kids don't get drunk, stoned, high, arrested, maimed, jailed, permanently injured or pregnant. Some do, but they are the minority. You decide whether you want to run with the majority or join the others. If you are 17 already, you are half way. Some researchers say that 17 is the year rational thought and sensible decision making starts to come to the fore, and by 25 you are fully adult.

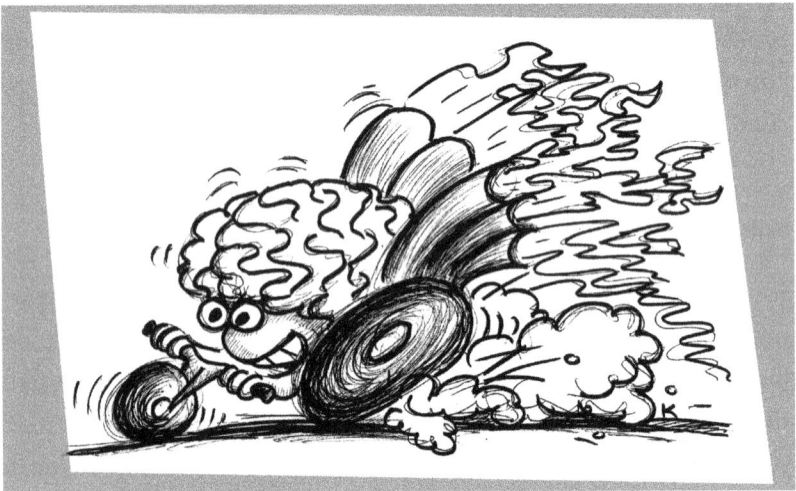

Video games

Video Games a risk? You think I've lost the plot? How can video games get teenagers drunk, stoned, high, arrested, maimed, jailed, permanently injured or pregnant? Well welcome again to the world of current brain research. There are dozens of research projects completed and underway on the effects of video games on young people.

First the good news: Video games aren't all bad. Psychologist Douglas Gentile finds some games are good for some people and professions. Surgeons who do operations using tiny video cameras and watching a screen may be better surgeons because of gaming. Air traffic controllers can sharpen their observation skills in screen watching.

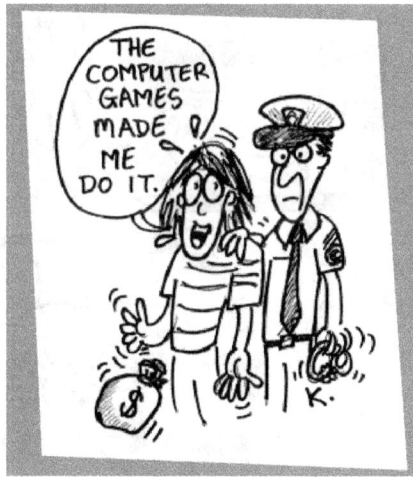

There are educational games which can help you master concepts you learn at school, and there are health programs which can teach children to manage problems better than their doctors can. Researchers also discovered that some games increased drivers' ability to see shades of grey – making them better night drivers. And there's good evidence that team games help people develop collaboration skills.

So, how can playing video games be a risky behaviour? Well, it depends on a number of factors, like how much time you spend playing them, the content of the game, whether you play alone or with friends etc. Dr Gentile says humans learn what they practice, and if a video games requires you to suppress your empathy or emotion or increase your level of violence, then you will. If you then become desensitised to virtual violence it's no big leap to be desensitized to actual violence. Having a 'violent brain' can lead to violent behaviour! Video games are risky if they lead to risky behaviour.

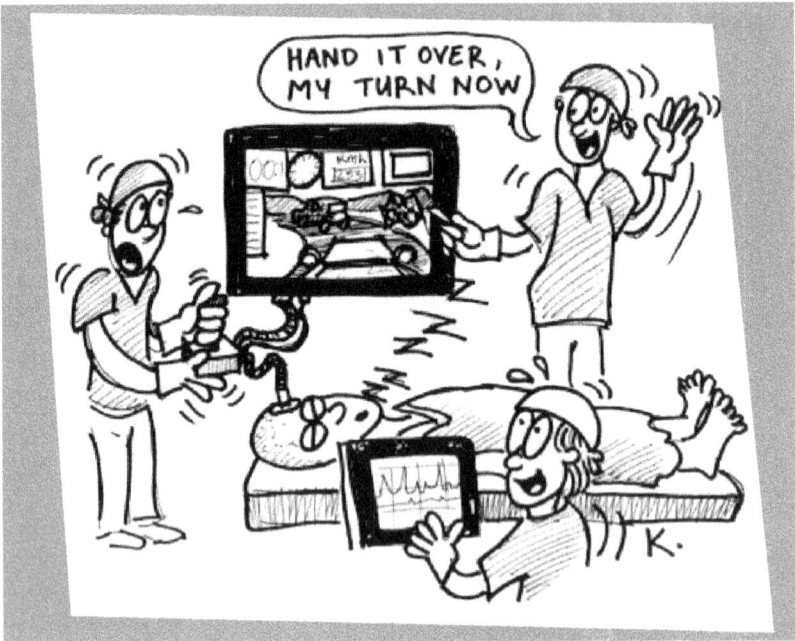

And while we're on video games: Many studies have found that school performance worsens in a direct correlation to increasing gaming time. No study has found the opposite! There's also an increased risk for keen gamers to become obese, less social and have other positive activities pushed to the back burner. Doctor and psychologist, Leonard Sax, reports that some young men are choosing video games over their friends, girlfriends or earning money.

Sax reports that several parts of the brain that work together for pleasure, reward, motivation and drive go 'out of kilter' in the brains of addicted game players. This can make it impossible for serious gamers to relate to the real world and thus they lose their motivation to lead a real life, instead finding their way only in the virtual world.

Scary stuff indeed! To avoid an addiction it helps to know two things: addiction is possible for some people, and you can make choices to avoid getting there.

These are decisions *you* have the power to make right now.

Bullying and Cyberbullying

Bullying is bad. Really bad. Don't put up with it. Just by being in a school, or on a computer, you are at risk, but there *are* things you can do about it if you, or someone you know, is being harassed by other people. And, if *you* are a bully then read the following carefully – you may be doing more harm than you realise.

The National Definition of Bullying for Australian Schools defines bullying as:

"an ongoing misuse of power in relationships through repeated verbal, physical and/or social behaviour that causes physical and/or psychological harm. It can involve an individual or a group misusing their power over one or more persons. Bullying can happen in person or online, and it can be obvious (overt) or hidden (covert).

Bullying of any form or for any reason can have long-term effects on those involved, including bystanders.

Single incidents and conflict or fights between equals, whether in person or online, are not defined as bullying

The new catchword, because we are so wired-up these days, is *cyberbullying*. This can be more than being teased in the playground or having your lunch money stolen, because cyber-bullying can be relentless. It continues at home, anytime someone logs on to a computer or phone. Sometimes people just never get a break – and that hurts, and they can find themselves spiralling down into depression and/or social withdrawal. Some people are even driven to harm themselves.

There are many ways you can be cyberbullied: through abusive texts or emails, via photos and videos (for example on Facebook, Snapchat etc), by having your identity stolen on line, being 'trolled' by gutless, anonymous bullies, being excluded, humiliated on line, through the use of 'revenge' porn, rumour mongering, nasty 'chatting' and so on.

If any of this is happening to you, then you want it stopped as soon as possible. You don't deserve it, you didn't ask for it, it is not your fault, and it must be stopped.

Firstly talk to someone you trust straight away. Your school will have a policy in place to address cyberbullying and your teachers will want to know of any instances immediately, no matter whether or not the bully is in your school. If there's nobody around call the Kids Help Line (1800 55 1800).

Remember a few simple rules: Always log off on school or public computers and never tell anyone your password. If cyberbullying comes your way, never retaliate or respond—they might use it against you – but also don't throw anything away. Cyberbullying in many cases is illegal, so keep texts and emails, and take screen shots of social networking conversations – they are evidence of someone else's wrong-doing.

You can also report abuse to the internet service, block the bully and change your privacy settings.

Your behaviour and your parents

Remember that in adolescence your prefrontal cortex, right at the front of your brain, is still being rewired. After adolescence you will think differently, plan more carefully, consider the consequences of your actions, and be less likely to take risks without weighing up the alternatives.

All teenagers, in fact all people, make mistakes. As a teen many of your mistakes are wonderful learning opportunities that mould you into the adult you will become. In your teens your parents need to pull back a little and allow you to make mistakes. Remember, their biology rules their behaviour as much as yours does, but we're all different, and some parents allow more freedom than others. Parents don't want you to make mistakes, but good parenting will allow you to get away with small ones and survive any big ones. And hopefully avoid the really big ones.

Your behaviour is the window through which your parents gauge how you're going and the level of responsibility they can allow you. Trying to understand their viewpoint will be tough for many teens, but it can open windows of opportunity you can't imagine until they are there.

Compare these three teens and think about their relationships with their parents. If you were a parent who would you trust more?

Mark is 17 and has his first car. He drives it fast and furiously, and has been caught doing burnouts in the neighbourhood. He smokes dope, and drinks and hangs out with, the boys outside the basketball stadium on Friday and Saturday nights. He steals money from his dad if he leaves it lying around, watches on-line porn, and has picked the easy subjects at a school which he plans to leave soon anyway. He is a (secret) virgin but has big plans with Laura once he gets rid of her boyfriend through intimidation.

Terry is 17 and wants to be a vet. He knows how many marks he needs in the exams and works to get them. He also plans on travelling overseas after the end of school, so cleans a laundry to earn money. He has a steady girlfriend, Laura, but they've agreed to wait until they're a bit older before having sex. He's a virgin and really looks forward to the day when he's not, but he's happy to wait for Laura. He rides a bicycle to school to save money and because it's greener. His major problem in life is bullying by Mark.

Laura is 16 and loves Terry deeply. She is not a virgin, but her only sexual experience was highly unsatisfactory, so she's in no hurry to repeat that. She and Terry will wait until everything is just perfect before going the whole way. She's thinking of joining him to go travelling after school finishes and is saving her money from her restaurant job and babysitting, just in case. Laura gets the attention of every boy at school, which she likes, as long as they leave her alone.

Okay okay, I set this up. One is a loser bully and two are the types of kids any parent would be proud of. These characters sound like they come from a cheap romance novel (maybe I'll write it some day), but they are based on real people I know.

If you were Mark, you're unlikely to be reading this book in the first place, but for a moment I want you to think about where Mark is likely to be when he's 25. What about Terry and Laura? Put yourself in their shoes. Who has the trust of their parents? Who has goals and knows how to achieve them? Who is happy?

You need to set goals during these years because soon you'll be adult and independent. One of the things you can do is look at people you know who are five or ten years older than you. What are they doing? How did they get there? Where are they likely to be in another five years? Are any of them role models you'd like to follow, or avoid? What do you want to do with your life?

Now, a note just for the young men: Family therapist and author Steve Biddulph, says in the current time many boys, especially, are lacking in adult male companionship and teaching because both fathers and the traditional uncle/grandfather/coach figure in your lives are too busy, or live too far away. In the past, male adults used to play bigger parts in the growth and development of young men, and these men were more likely than not to be someone other than the boy's father. Many societies have, or had, initiation rites into manhood and perhaps they're a sad loss to many modern cultures. Your development into an adult is unstoppable, but it's important that you are taught how to be a man by successful, trustworthy and appropriate adult men. You need to find such men to help you and avoid being led by guys who are as confused about their manhood as most teens are. This way can lead to wasted years and destruction.

While I am talking to the guys – a note about pornography: many doctors and neuroscientists like Doidge, are reporting negative effects on the brains of young men who are accessing massive amounts of free porn via the internet and becoming addicted. Sax says that in some areas the *major* sexual relationship young men are having is with graphic digital images. Because sexual release produces your 'feel good' hormones, pornography can be addictive. Any addiction is a problem, so be aware. And if you are choosing to sit alone, at your computer, rather than chat up girls, then you may have a problem – talk to your school counsellor or trusted adult friend if you think you do. There are girls out there wondering what's wrong… where are all the boys?

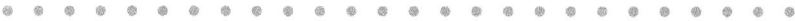

THINK ABOUT IT

* What are the major risks you take? Are they 'perceived risks' or real?
* Are there any risks you are now taking that you'd like to avoid? How would you go about this? (If you need help, see the back of this book for more information.)

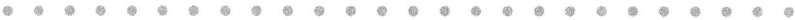

A MESSAGE TO YOUR TEACHERS

When I was at school we were allowed to climb trees and play *Red Rover*, both potentially dangerous activities. Everyone I know survived these 'risks' and more, despite a few injuries.

Modern schools have more rules than most armies or prisons. There is more you can't do than can, and schools are frightened of litigation for negligence. Teachers have to be more responsible than the average parent, because they are trained professionals, and no one has a degree in parenting. The appetite teens have for adventure and risk has not changed over the years and schools these days, perhaps by default, have to engineer opportunities for their students' growth in this area.

Many schools offer 'outreach' programs like camping or bush walking, and other activities, which kids might not experience otherwise. The best I have heard of recently is a bunch of year 8 middle school kids riding Bactrian camels overland for a week in Mongolia! Wow!

Activities like these are very positive influences on the learning and growth of teenagers and, in Brain Compatible Education terms, they are powerful 'episodic learning events' because of their multi-sensory nature. Special, safe learning opportunities, with high emotional input, are remembered long after the average school lesson.

Effective teaching happens through a variety of methodologies. School field trips are particularly effective and they can offer excitement and perceived risks that teenagers will benefit from greatly.

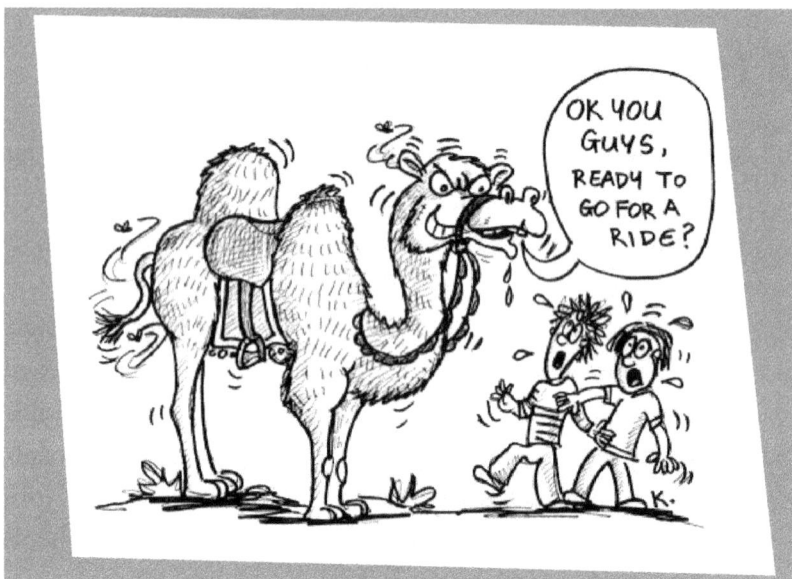

A MESSAGE TO YOUR PARENTS

Your kids are growing in a society addicted to the media. The media focuses on sex and drugs and every day thousands of images of the 'perfect' girlfriend, or boyfriend, might be presented to your son or daughter. Few of us measure up to the figures portrayed and even fewer of us are doing what they're doing. Most kids are *not* taking drugs, having wild sex, getting drunk, and car surfing or otherwise endangering their lives. Some are, and because of this, parenting is a worry.

We need to be there for our kids and allow them to take risks, explore the world and identify their own place in it. They will make mistakes, but we can help them pick up the pieces and build up their resilience to the knocks and bruises of life.

Remember the perceived risk of the roller coaster? That's all it needs. Many kids need to think they're taking big risks; it's a part of growing up. But real risks, where they endanger their lives or health, or other people, need to be avoided. In my opinion one of the things parents must do at all costs is die before their kids (at a ripe old age, of course). That's the natural order, nothing to me could be worse than burying my own child.

So our job is to protect our children, all the while allowing them to build their independence, so they too can make their own way in the world. Most of us do this without a problem, but nobody ever said it was going to be easy.

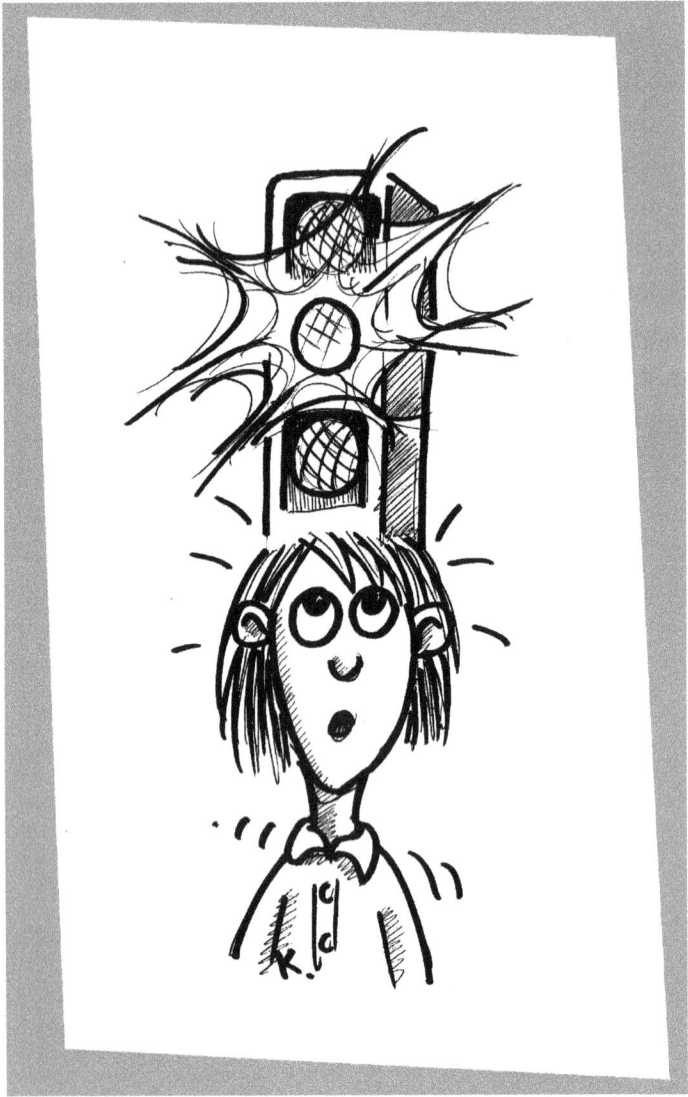

Chapter 11

Stress

. . . .

IN THIS CHAPTER YOU WILL LEARN
* How stress can be good for you.
* How stress can be bad for you.

. . . .

*E*verybody experiences stress. Short bursts of acute stress are normal and stress is important. It sharpens your attention and hones your skills. You can easily imagine the importance of stress for our early ancestors. The flight or fight response, activated by the hormones adrenalin and cortisol (see Chapter 8), allows you to rapidly escape, or defend yourself, from wild animal attacks.

These days few of us live on the plains of Africa, so low levels of stress can be used to improve your performance at school, on the sports field, and even in arguments with friends or parents. This stress fades away quickly and leaves no permanent imprint on you. Trouble arises if you are under constant high levels of stress. Teenagers may experience ongoing problems that put them under such stress.

Constant or chronic stress may be caused by school bullies, domineering parents or siblings, sexual predators, poverty, drugs (yours or other peoples'), boyfriend/girlfriend issues, fear for personal safety, not enough sleep, or confusion about what's happening.

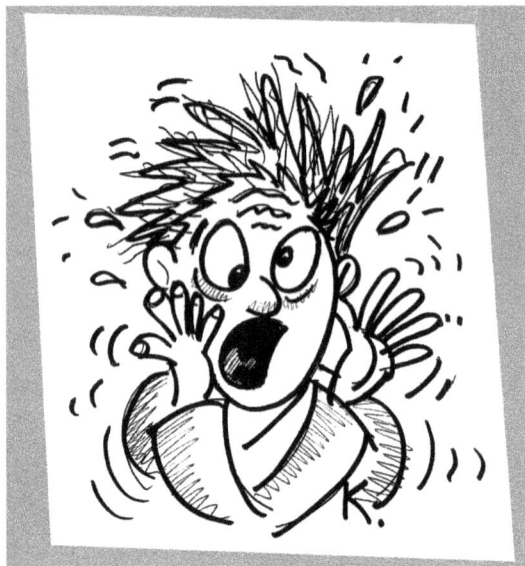

Chronic stress can be an ongoing torture and it can have permanent effects on your body and brain. For instance, it can cause a raised level of blood sugar, which can lead to a rise in the hormone that metabolises sugar, insulin. If this goes on for too long it can lead to Type 2 diabetes.

FUN FACT:
STRESS CAN BE HANDY
FOR A BURST OF
EXTRA ENERGY AND
CONCENTRATION, LIKE
WHEN YOU'RE COMPETING
OR SITTING AN EXAM.

Your normal stable self may no longer cope, and may have to change, in an attempt to reach a new stability. This process is known as *allostasis*. The change will come at a price, which scientists call the allostatic load. Your body pays, because it is less efficient or overwhelmed, and it needs to expend energy to maintain a stable system.

Problems that affect the mental and physical health of people arise when the systems involved in allostasis don't shut off when they're not needed. Or they don't become active when they are needed. Or the problem goes on for so long, the higher or lower levels become normal.

People under chronic stress may exhibit some or all of the following symptoms: constant sickness from a weakened immune system; high blood pressure; poor memory (your hippocampus may actually shrivel up); obesity; low sex drive, hardened arteries. Chronic stress seems to eat you up. It dampens your ability to keep track of information by impairing the excitement of nerve cells. You must do something to counteract it, and fortunately this may not be too hard

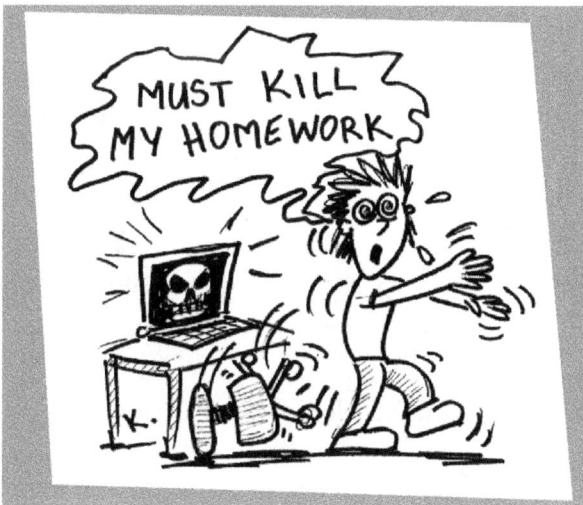

Killing chronic stress

Chronic stress can be fought by a number of simple tactics. Firstly try relaxing. Work out whatever soothes you best – music, meditation, walks on the beach, hobbies, whatever, and *actively* use these activities to calm down. Spending time with friends and laughing helps greatly. Exercise, or any form of aerobic activity, can help you relax too (see Chapter 4). Exercise pumps the blood around more. This removes toxins and cortisol from your brain. A fit person with a fit brain is clearly more prepared to learn.

Remember cortisol is soluble in water, so always be well hydrated (with water, not sugary drinks).

FUN FACT:
CONTINUOUS STRESS
CHANGES THE SIZE,
STRUCTURE AND
FUNCTIONING OF YOUR
BRAIN.

You also need to feel safe and unthreatened. If you are not in a safe environment then try to do something about it. Seek help and counselling if this is hard. Think of problems as challenges rather than disasters. You can always tackle challenges, but disasters can be a disaster! Work out in your mind what is valuable. Don't worry too much about trivial things or the things you can't change, and expect to make mistakes.

Building up your resilience to mistakes, and to the blows of living, will help you to bounce back faster. You can do this in part by forgiving yourself if you make a mistake, and moving on. Also by taking control of your life, being honest to yourself, and learning to be assertive.

And you *must* sleep, and have lots of it (see Chapter 3). As a teenager you'll need about nine or ten hours each night on average. Getting a good night's sleep would possibly solve the problems of many teenagers around the world.

There is also good scientific evidence that meditation lowers stress and, in fact, meditation actually promotes the growth of grey matter and delays the effects of aging – just ask the Dalai Lama.

And if all this isn't enough, try one of the strongest stress relievers around: help someone else. This is known as altruism. Lots of people, from the elderly, to those with disabilities, the sick and the infirm, would find life easier if more of us were willing to help. Being altruistic makes you feel better about yourself and more in control, so stress is lowered. And think about this mantra: it puts things into perspective for me:

'I used to complain I had no shoes, until I met a man who had no feet.'

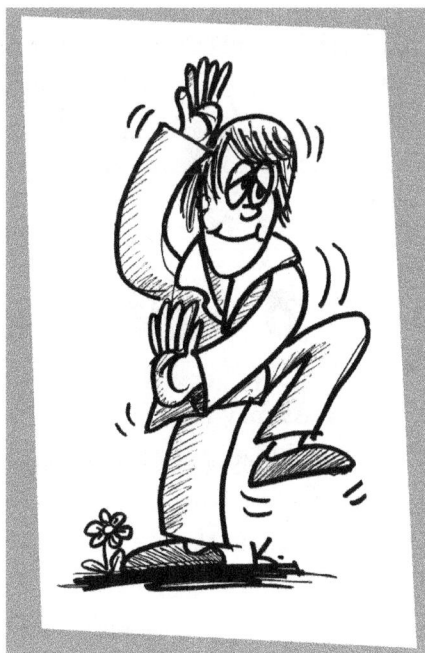

- -

THINK ABOUT IT

* List the major stresses in your life right now?
* If you can identify them perhaps you can work out a plan to lessen them.
* Is there someone who can help you (a school counsellor, grand parent, parent, friend)?
* Remember there are counsellors ready to talk to you on the phone 24 hours a day, for example:

Kids Help Line ph 1800 55 1800 and
Beyond Blue ph 1300 22 4636.
(See the back of this book for more information.)

- -

A MESSAGE TO YOUR TEACHERS

Teenagers in your class may be stressed by many things – for example: exams; workload; unrealistic classroom demands; disagreements with you or other adults; the death or illness of friends or family or a pet; an abusive or neglectful home life: or by a combination of many things. They may also have boyfriend or girlfriend problems, difficulties with bullies, and concerns about their physical appearance and development.

Any situation where they, or even their loved ones, are under physical or emotional threats may cause stress to such a degree that achieving your lesson plan learning objectives will seem unlikely. I was Principal of a school which catered for the children of air force personnel when the Gulf War broke out and the squadron was deployed to Iraq. Almost immediately we had to soothe fears and counsel students, and also some teachers who were wives of air force personnel, who were sure their fathers or husbands were about to be killed. School work was irrelevant when compared to these fears and it was a reminder of how some learning will only take place after more important things are dealt with.

Some kids might also live in dread that they'll be called upon by you to answer questions in public, as they might have a mind-numbing fear of public speaking or losing face in class. Teachers need to take all these things into account and develop strategies to help. Scaffolding of the processes required might be needed. For example, public speaking can move from reading texts to supporting notes as confidence increases. When I was at school I used to shake badly when forced to public speaking. Even at university I used to continue to tremble with fear in front of an audience, but now I am a professional speaker, which I marvel at, when I remember my teenage self.

If you are unsure about how to help stressed students, don't go it alone. Speak to the school counsellor or other staff if there is a problem.

Also get trained in, or read up on, brain compatible learning techniques, and vary your methods of delivery of material. Students will struggle less as you will cater for individual learning styles more.

A MESSAGE TO YOUR PARENTS

Do you contribute to your teenager's stress? It's most likely you do, they certainly contribute to yours. Teenagers require boundaries that keep them safe and healthy. Some require more boundaries than others of course, but consider those that you impose on your kids. Are any of them unreasonable? Remember in these years your kids will need to start accepting responsibility for their actions and the sooner they do, the better, but they need to be allowed to.

If you come from a large family you may have been dismayed if you were the eldest (or surprised if you're the youngest) over your parents relaxing rules over the years. Parents seem to routinely adjust their parenting as the youngest grows up, perhaps because they become more expert at it with experience. In my own family my big brother and I were always amazed at how different life was for our youngest brother and sister.

My point is that many parents might relax a little more if they take the time to evaluate what's important about their relationships with the kids, and stop 'sweating the small stuff'.

There are a number of excellent books listed at the back of this book about parenting teenagers. Every parent can learn more about parenting.

Chapter 12

Girls and Boys ARE Different!

● ●

IN THIS CHAPTER YOU WILL LEARN

✳ That there are differences between the brains of males and females.

✳ Ten parts of the brain you can easily identify.

● ●

Have you ever wondered why many of the girls you know like Facebook, or gossip magazines, while many of the boys watch YouTube and read magazines about cars, or soccer, instead? If I say the words "chick flick" to you, do you just *know* the type of movie I mean and who is most likely to enjoy it? Do the boys you know prefer to kick a football with their mates, or sit around chatting, doing each other's hair and nails?

Well, for most of the last fifty years what I am going to say now was an uncomfortable thing to say: GIRLS AND BOYS HAVE DIFFERENT BRAINS. Now we can shout it from the rooftops, but people used to whisper it as, even though everyone could see obvious male and female traits, it was not politically correct to talk about them. In those days there was much arguing over the equality of the sexes and people dared not declare one gender's brain was different to the other because others would immediately assume this meant 'better' or 'smarter'. Nowadays we know that one is *not* better than the other, even though there really are distinct differences.

For decades there was the great 'nature verses nurture' debate. Some people used to say that boys' and girls' brains were hardwired into having girl traits or boy traits which meant what you have you are born with. Others would claim that girls and boys are the same at birth and that girls became girly because they are given dolls to play with and pink bedrooms, while boys receive toy trains and trucks in their blue painted rooms. Most scientists used to have a foot in both camps and say yes, we are different at birth, but it's how we are treated and our life experiences that turn us into the gender we present.

FUN FACT:
A SCIENTIST COULD
NOT TELL IF A
BRAIN WAS MALE OR
FEMALE WITHOUT A
DNA CHECK.

Well, careful research and technology changed all that. For example the functional magnetic resonance imaging (fMRI) machine can scan the brains of males and females of all ages whilst their owners are alive and thinking and doing simple tasks. They can actually watch what is happening in the brain, where it's taking place, and measure how much energy is involved. As more research is done, more differences between male and female brains become distinctly obvious.

A word of warning here: It is possible for males to show female brain patterns and for females to show male brain patterns. It does not detract from your masculinity or femininity, nor does it have anything to do with homosexuality or heterosexuality. I wish there were better terms for brains other than 'male' or 'female' in this context because they are more *tendencies* or averages than hard classifications, but through the work of researchers like Dr Simon Baron-Cohen, a professor of Developmental Psychopathology in the UK, these terms are now well known.

If you are a male who happens to feel that the colour of your mobile phone is important (possibly a female trait) or a girl who is more interested in the number of megapixels in the phone camera or the RAM (possibly a more male trait) then good for you. Please do not read into this Chapter anything more than that – preferences like these do not affect your sexuality or your value as a human being. They are, in fact, what makes each of us unique and interesting people.

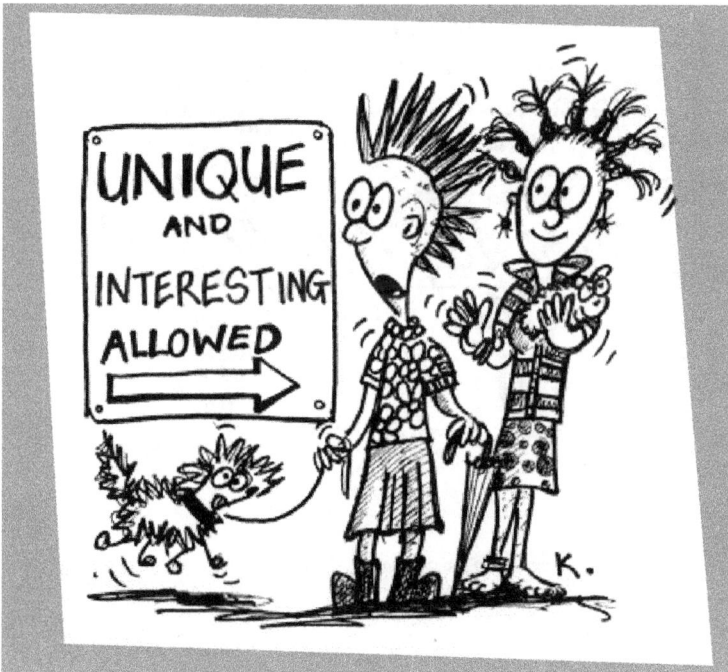

If we were to dissect a bunch of brains of both male and females what would we discover?

Well, it would be very difficult to tell whether an unlabelled brain was male, female, homosexual or transgender, and we'd need a really big pile to be able to average our measurements. But if we were sure of the brain's gender and we could measure hundreds of brains, we'd firstly see that the *average* male brain is bigger than the average female brain. No surprise here, average males also have bigger heads and bodies too, but brain size has little effect on intelligence. The only thing we can say for sure about people with big heads is that they wear big hats.

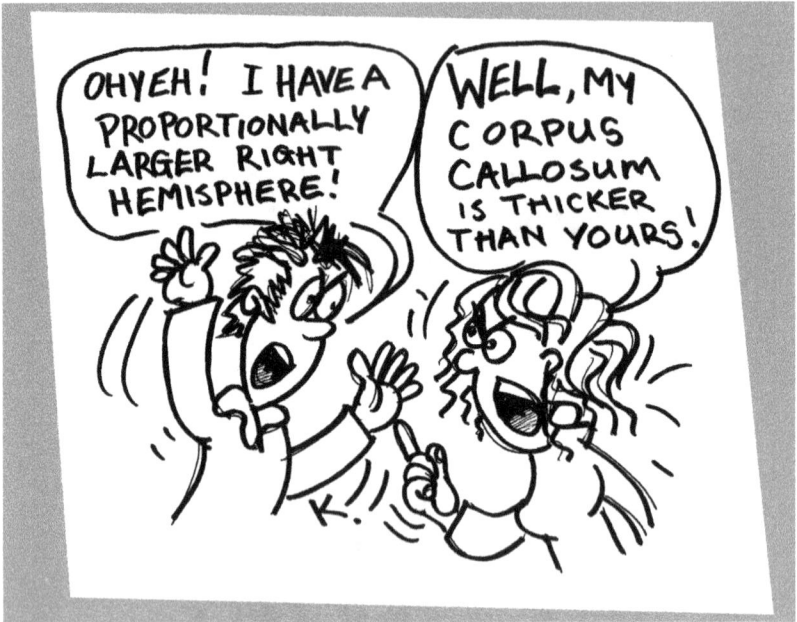

We would also find that females often have more symmetrical brains, whilst males have a proportionally larger right hemisphere.

The corpus callosum (the part of the brain that joins the left side and the right side, allowing billions of neurons to connect the hemispheres) is thicker in females than in males. Perhaps this is because girls use both sides of the brain when communicating, while males tend to use the left side more.

Different parts of the brain grow at different rates in males and females. Teenage males have faster growing amygdala, but the girls have a faster growing hippocampus and larger basal ganglia. Boys have a larger cerebellum. Big differences? Perhaps not, but remember what these parts do. Your amygdala runs your fight or flight response system, your emotions and 'gut' reactions. Your basal ganglia allow smoother functioning of your frontal cortex, which is important in judgement and 'sensible' thinking. Your hippocampus is important for memory and your cerebellum for physical coordination.

But why are there differences? Most writers on this topic think they are something to do with our evolution – when our ancestors were more affected by the 'survival of the fittest' rules than we appear to be in the modern world. Males and females came under different selection pressures, so certain male and female traits evolved if they were of advantage to the person, in terms of the numbers and survival of their babies. Men had to hunt and therefore needed the stamina and physical strength to bring back the meat. Women did most of the child rearing and needed to stay closer to the children, so were more productive in the gathering of plant foods than the men. As for the evolution of our language abilities, you can imagine early men grunting to each other with few words on the hunt, whilst the women gossiped around the home area. Perhaps little has changed.

Dr Baron-Cohen says the main difference between the average male and female brain is that males tend to analyse and construct systems and females tend to empathise. His theory goes on to describe how brain disorders, such as autism, are really just the appearance of *hyper*-male brains which can be very good at systemising but poor at empathising.

All this means teenage boys are the ones most likely to *want* to quote sports statistics, read maps, dismantle cars and motor bikes, and put them back together again, skip stones and throw javelins. Girls can do all those things too, but most don't want to, so they don't practise the skills. Instead, girls are more likely to use language. They spend more time with close friends, talking on the phone, on-line chatting and generally being more sociable. They like shopping, eat better foods, take fewer risks and don't worry so much about fine details or statistics. You can see these differences in the choices teenagers make in school subjects. More boys take on physics and maths, girls like English and social studies. This is reflected in the relative sizes of the appropriate brain parts in the *average* boy or girl. If you are a girl who excels in maths and physics, or a boy who is a great writer or you love ballet, then make the most of your talents.

FUN FACT: THE AVERAGE MALE BRAIN IS BIGGER THAN THE AVERAGE FEMALE BRAIN, BUT SIZE DOES NOT NECESSARILY AFFECT INTELLIGENCE. EINSTEIN'S BRAIN WAS SMALLER THAN AVERAGE.

The differences can be negative too. Boys are more likely to be criminals than girls so there are many more males than females in prison. They are also more likely to stutter and have language problems like dyslexia, and other brain disorders such as autism, and Asperger's Syndrome. Girls are more prone to suffering depression and having eating disorders.

Testosterone and oestrogen

For teenagers like you, the effects of the sex hormones, testosterone and oestrogen, on your bodies through the teenage years after puberty are obvious. They are turning you from a child to adult – changing your body shape, enlarging some important parts, giving you body hair and deeper voices. These outward changes are as much about making you attractive to the opposite sex, as preparing you to take on adult roles such as finding food, providing shelter and rearing babies, but they may take a number of years to come into effect.

Testosterone is the male sex hormone and oestrogen the female, though we all have some of each and both of them are made in your gonads – either testicles or ovaries, depending on your gender.

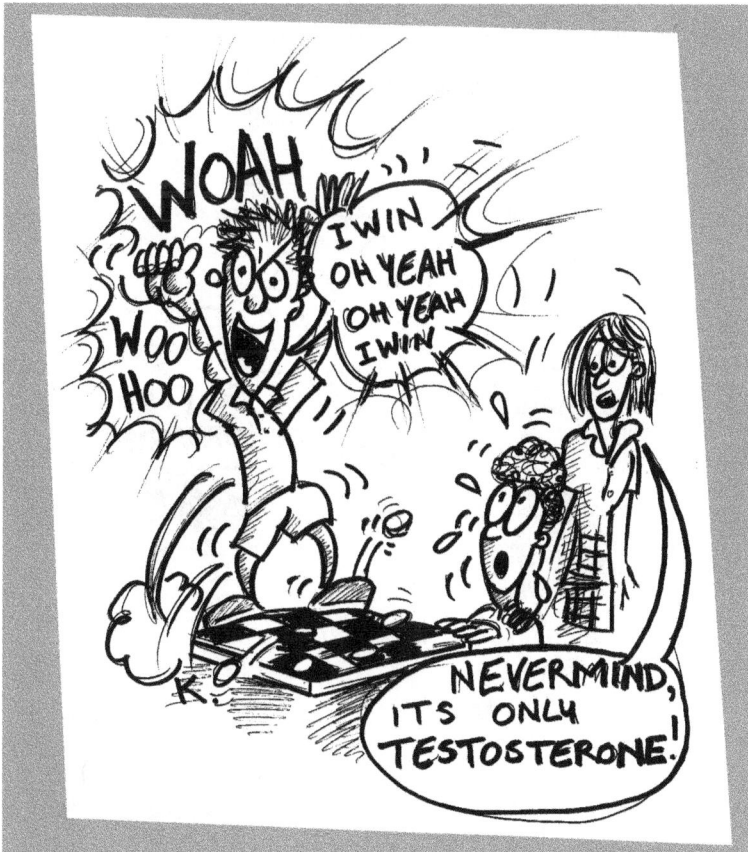

The effect of these hormones on your brain is also important. Testosterone is linked to aggression – the more you have the higher it is. You get a burst of it when you're playing sport – especially if you're winning.

Oestrogen promotes more active brain cells and alertness so higher levels of it might lead to increased learning. Of course, oestrogen plays the major role in regulating a woman's menstrual cycle, so it's higher at some times of the cycle than others. It also can affect dopamine levels. You read in Chapter 8 that dopamine usually makes you feel great, but sometimes it can tip you into a foul mood. Some, though not all, women become moody during parts of their menstrual cycles, and it's likely to be related to hormonal changes. Moodiness affects the ability to learn as well.

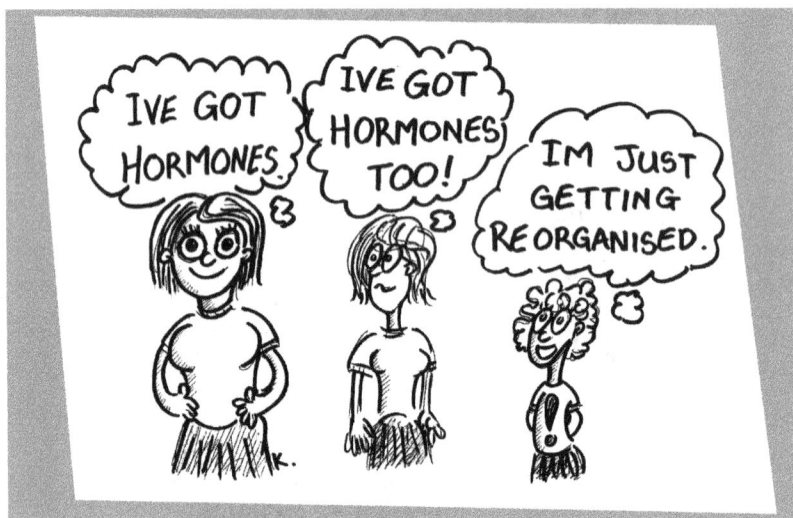

Have I repeated the main message of this Chapter enough?

Yes, there are differences between the brains of males and females. Evolution would suggest that this must have been very necessary in our species' history. Humans are a very successful species, so any differences we have are likely to have been important in human survival and perhaps essential in bringing the sexes together. The differences do not reflect intelligence or superiority and they are differences seen mainly in averages, anyway. We all have traits that on any scale would be seen as more feminine and others that would be seen as more masculine. Plus, as you already know, you can train your brain to learn anything you want it to.

A MESSAGE TO YOUR TEACHERS

The differences between male and female brains are slowly being unravelled. As educators we need to avoid stereotyping and not label all boys or girls as male brained or female brained because individuals may be far from the average. Some boys will have female brain traits and some girls will have male brain traits. But, considering what neuroscientists and psychologists have discovered about sex differences of *average* brains what effects can this knowledge have on how we teach our students?

Neuroscientists like Dr Denckla, at The Kennedy Krieger Institute, are saying that some of the differences we see at school may be related to different maturation ages in different parts of the brain. In boys the areas needed for maths, spatial relationships (geometry) appear to be maturing four years earlier than in girls. In girls the language and fine motor skills, such as those needed for handwriting, appear up to six years ahead of boys. This may mean an average twelve year old girl has a maths brain like an eight year old boy but a language brain like an eighteen year old boy. Yale University researchers discovered that females also use more of their brain in communication – parts of both hemispheres light up in an fMRI scan of communicating women, but males tend to use only one side, usually the left hemisphere.

One more word about the maths ability of boys: as neuroscientists Aamodt and Wang point out, it's true that many boys top the scores in maths, but there are also more at the other end of the scale. Males are more variable than females and although the difference is small, it looms large in the life of individuals who are a long way from the average – either way.

Most teachers have anecdotes and observations of their students that seem to agree with this research, although, of course, there are many exceptions.

Information such as this will help teachers to program for, and use, brain compatible education techniques with their students. Girls are likely to succeed to a higher level in maths if it is more social – for example through group work, discussion, relationship based education. Boys can be helped with their language use by teaching through more systemised processes, studying 'male topics' such as machinery and sports and giving opportunities to talk and write about them.

Our male and female students deserve equal opportunities and we need to be continually promoting gender equality within our schools, including any LGBTQ individuals. But because males and females develop at different rates and have different strengths, treating them the same may not be giving equal opportunity. As Eric Jenson says in *Brain Based Learning*, "Let's acknowledge differences; and work with boys and girls in ways that best match their own developmental and learning needs".

And *why not* teach according to how the brains learn?

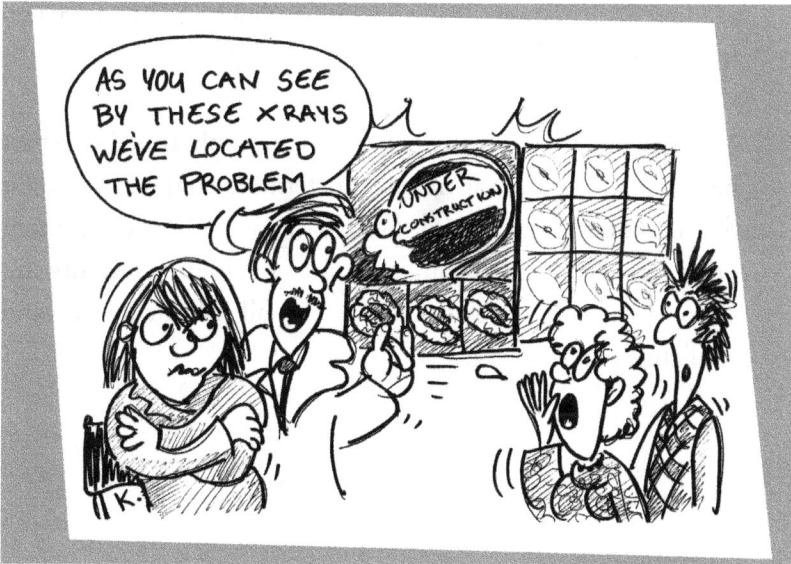

A MESSAGE TO YOUR PARENTS

We all know about the differences between the sexes. It didn't take long in my married life for me to learn that going shopping with my wife was an endurance test. She *never* wants to spend time in the hardware store, or camping shops and will pick through a hundred fruit to find the best five in the grocer's. There's nothing wrong with the way she shops, it just drives me up the wall. I drank three coffees in a cafe once, waiting for her in the shoe-shop next door. And she didn't even buy anything!

Whether you are the parent of boys or girls, the 'nature verses nurture' debate is still of interest. We may well have encouraged our children's gender stereotyping by buying dolls for our daughters and planes for our sons. And we possibly have often excused our children's behaviour because of their gender when we say things like "boys will be boys" or "*girls* don't do that!"

New research in neuroscience has shown the physical differences between the brains of males and females that lead to their different gender traits, and there's little we can do about them, other than accept them, and promote our children's talents and support them in their weaknesses. It's all part of the joy and challenge of parenting.

Chapter 13

Choices

- -

IN THIS CHAPTER YOU WILL LEARN

* That the road to your identity and your future may be bumpy
* There are many things you can do to prepare yourself for your future.

- -

Who are you? What are you good at? What will you do with your life?

Your teenage years are the years when you further develop answers to these questions. Much of what you go through is teaching you about yourself, and the person you can be as an adult. I don't mean just your future career or profession, but your personal identity. In his Teen Survival Guide, *Yes, Your Parents Are Crazy*, psychologist Dr Michael Bradley says "...developing your identity means trying on a million hats of ideas and values, to see which ones fit you". Make no mistake; the ride can be bumpy, filled with experiences, disappointments and frustrations you would rather do without. But there are also wonderful, exciting things that happen. Your brain is developing fast, these are your peak learning years and the changes can be exciting and challenging, and proof that you are growing up.

There are two important things to remember about your identity journey. First, you are not alone. Other teenagers are going through it too, and all adults have been there. They may not remember how confusing, frustrating or hard it can be, but if you need help and you know someone you can trust, talk to him or her, and seek support. Secondly, although to you the teen years may seem to be unending, in the grand scheme of your life, they're actually over very quickly. What you go through as you morph into an adult is important and the choices you make now can affect your life for a very long time.

Help yourself

The best education is that which empowers the learner to help themselves. You've read this far, so now you have some more knowledge that will give you confidence to make good choices.

For example, there are ways you can choose to change your moods. Changing moods is just shifting from the down hormones to the up hormones.

The best way of all is sleep. You're a teenager. Statistics say you get nine hours *less* sleep a week now than I did as a kid in the 1970s. You could be sleep deprived. Read Chapter 3 on the importance of sleep again. *If you do nothing else, to improve your mood, get your sleep patterns right.* Sleep also improves your learning and you're more likely to stay out of trouble.

Poor light might be affecting you. In the classroom, move closer to the window to be in natural light. Keep the house lights dim in the evening, and don't sit too close to the TV! Sleep in the dark. Blue light can directly affect your pineal gland which makes melatonin, the hormone of sleep. (Perhaps an incorrect level of melatonin, from the effects of blue light, helps you play a video game until dawn without feeling tired.)

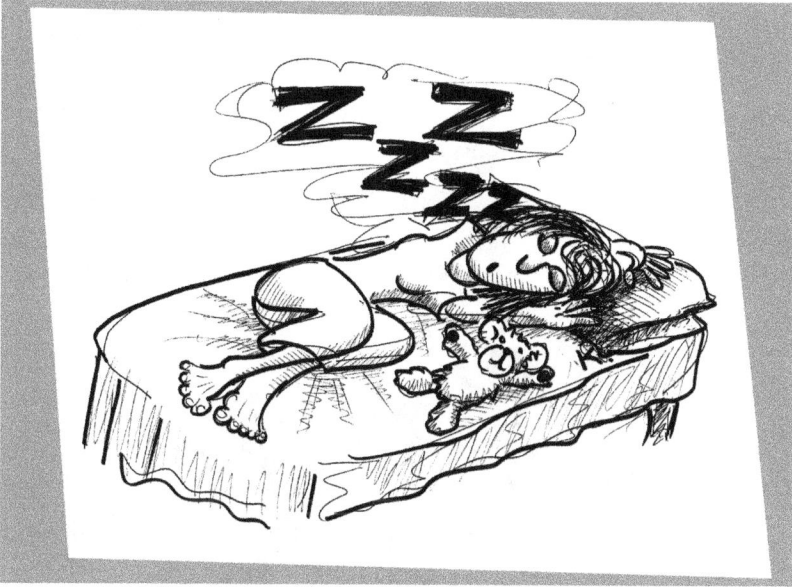

You already know that computer or videogames can be fun and you develop a lot of skills playing them (though many may be skills of little use outside the virtual world). Some games are social – they're what you talk about with your mates, you may even play against your friends in a virtual world. They are therefore part of your sense of self. However, you can and should make a conscious decision about how important they are to you, and how to get a balance between screen-based and real life activities.

If *you* self-limit the time you spend on your phone, TV, movies, and computers then you'll feel better about it than if you're having family fights about them. They are often sources of great fun and entertainment, but they can suck you in and cause you to spend countless unproductive hours on screens.

Music can affect you too. Listen to nicer music – you *know* what I mean. It can really affect your mood. Or better still, play an instrument. I learned the harmonica when I was 19 so I could play when out camping – corny I know, but I still have a lot of fun with it, and playing it always cheers me up.

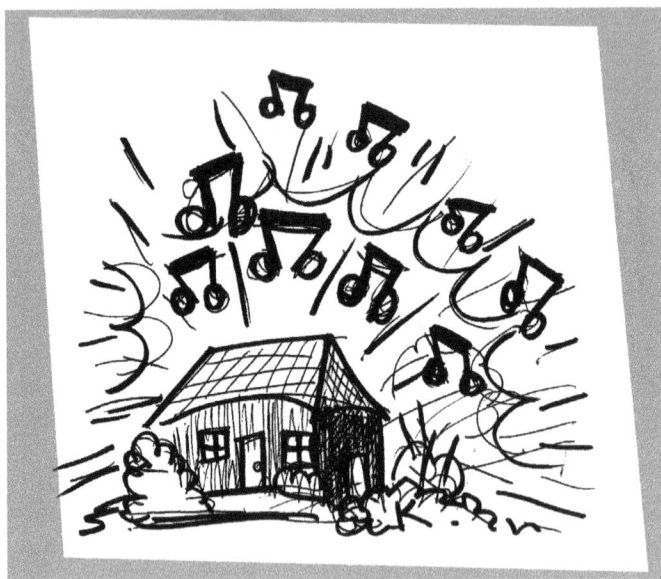

Ask your friends not to text or phone you when you need to be asleep. If the phone is a problem leave it outside the bedroom or turn it off. Don't allow yourself to be woken without a good reason.

Make things right with your family. Really shock them one day by telling them you love them – this is not easy for many teenagers, especially boys.

Most parents are doing the best they can, knowing what they know. Their apprenticeship was their own childhood. No one has a degree in parenting; we all learn it as we go along. Trust that you're loved, even if it doesn't feel like it sometimes. Your parents are, after all, governed by the same hormones as you, so they have a biological necessity to love their children. It's wired into their brains!

FUN FACT:
THE HUMAN BRAIN
IS THE ONLY ORGAN
THAT HAS NAMED
ITSELF.

If you've read all this, and you're having trouble making enough serotonin and dopamine even after talking with your friends, laughing, changing your diet, or following the other tips in this book, or if you just feel bad all the time, you'll worry about it less if you get help. You are not alone – lots of teenagers feel this way and lots of adults devote their lives to helping them get through it. So talk to a trusted family member; your doctor; a parent of a friend that you admire; your school counsellor or someone you trust and know cares about you. If they can't help, maybe they'll know someone who can. Never give in and never give up. See the back of this book for easy to make contacts with trained counsellors who can help.

Your learning and career profile

You will have noticed that your classmates are not the same as you. Some are academic, and love books and studying. For some school is a breeze and they seem to sail through it without working overly hard. Some prefer anything else in life other than school and spend their class time gossiping, passing notes or standing outside in the corridor. Some like sports, others join the chess club. Some will be involved in all the drama productions, others prefer rock climbing. Your preferences in things like these are personal and individual, and can be termed as your *interest profile*. When you really enjoy learning something that you are interested in, it seems almost effortlessness.

But not all learning is like that. Even things you are good at can take a lot of time and effort to learn.

Learning happens in four stages:

Acquisition: being aware and initial processing, Short-Term Memory

Rehearsal: practising, Working Memory

Retention: consolidating, Long-Term Memory

Retrieval: use and modification, Recall

Each person has a set of preferences for how they prefer to Acquire and Rehearse. For example, if your science project was to study the life cycle of frogs, would you prefer to use the internet to get the information, or to build an aquarium and observe and record changes over time?

Of course, your *learning profile*, which shows your preferences for various learning methods, may not be the most *efficient* way to learn something. It is probably more efficient to learn about frogs through reading about them on the internet, but for many of us, nowhere near as much fun, and nowhere near as memorable as mucking about in an aquarium or a pond.

When you go to school, teachers generally try to take account of class preferences within a framework of efficiency because there is just so much to get through. If the teacher's preferences are the direct opposite of yours, and the content is meaningless for you, school can become a daily drudge! Knowing your learning profile helps you to understand why some students connect with school, while others, equally smart and capable, reject it. Even more important, knowing your leaning profile enables you to learn without a teacher present! It builds your independence as a learner and your belief in your capacity to learn.

Imagine for a moment that you are in your mid-thirties and working full time... What job are you doing? What learning did you have to do to get that job? Learning doesn't stop when you leave school, it is a life-long process, and every time you change career there will be some new learning involved. Your learning profile can suggest occupations and career choices that you are most interested in, or most suited to. Even better, once you have a range of career choices in your mind, a learning profile can assist you to identify the areas to develop in order to reach your goals, and a plan for how to get there.

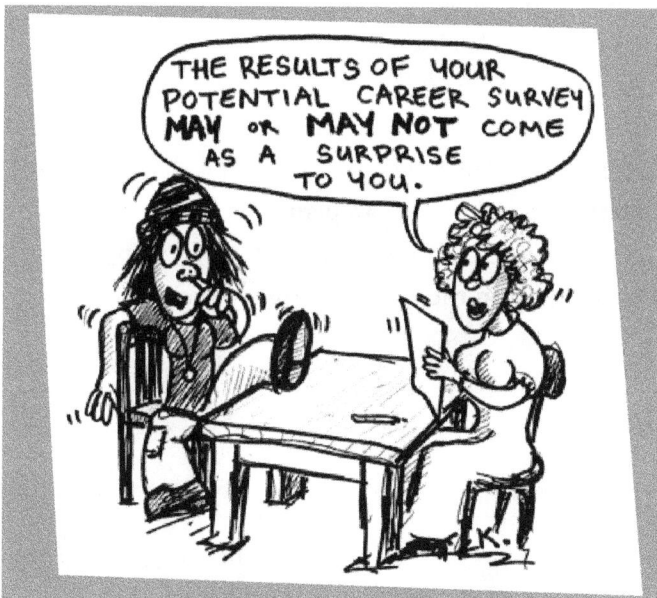

There are a number of 'personality' tests or career surveys around you may have seen, and your school may have got you to complete some. If you haven't, and are interested, go and see your school careers counsellor as soon as possible.

A last word on schools

School works well for most students, most of the time. However, success in classrooms is often a poor indicator of success beyond classrooms. It's hard to see it from the classroom, but even the bored or troublesome can, and do, reach greatness. Here are comments from two of the greatest:

"The only time my education was interrupted was while I was at school." – Winston Churchill.

"Education is what remains when one has forgotten everything one learnt at school." – Albert Einstein.

The adult world is packed with high flyers who did not do well, or who did not reach their potential at school. If you can recognise your talents, or a niche, you can plan for a future that is dependent more on your interests, talents and effort, than your connectedness to school. If you plan the future you really want, then you may just get it.

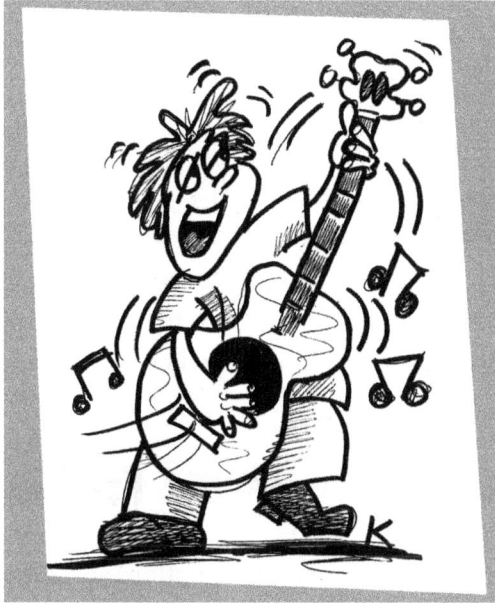

THINK ABOUT IT

* Note down two or three goals or ideas you have for your future. For example careers or jobs you are interested in, your plans. Write a 'bucket list' of things to do.
* What can you do this year to help achieve these goals?

A MESSAGE TO YOUR TEACHERS

Your students will need help to choose appropriate pathways. In high schools, often, there is a school careers counsellor who will help, but some will come and see you too. One of the joys of teaching is the help we can give young people at this important time of life. Our role as teachers is to be available, and ready to offer support and advice, if and when it is needed. Good luck.

A MESSAGE TO YOUR PARENTS

Each child's schooling and career options are shaped by a variety of influences. Significantly, these influences include: ability, motivation, confidence, strategies, strengths and interests.

Parents are their children's first and most significant teachers and mentors. It is parents who hold unconditional positive regard for their kids, and it is parents who gain the greatest degree of satisfaction from seeing their children identify, adjust and develop their capabilities. Teenagers have the right to make their own choices, but our role as a parent can be an important one. Our sons and daughters will need support and encouragement.

Chapter 14
Other Brains

· ·

IN THIS CHAPTER YOU WILL LEARN

✴ Some of the different brains you may encounter

· ·

Most teenagers have *normal* brains, but what normal means is a matter of debate, because every brain is different. Nevertheless there are brain conditions that we will call 'not normal'. You should know about these. When you meet people who have these differences, a little understanding of what they are going through will help develop your tolerance and empathy.

FUN FACT:
THERE IS ALMOST NO DIFFERENCE IN BRAIN ANATOMY BETWEEN THOSE PEOPLE WITH AUTISM AND THOSE WITHOUT IT.

This chapter summarises the more common conditions and a few things that may go wrong. You have probably heard of depression, ADD, ADHD, and ODD and it's likely you even know kids who have been diagnosed with these conditions. In fact, these conditions are common enough to seem 'normal' in today's society, and if we view them as challenges to be overcome, rather than disabilities, we will display more tolerance and compassion for the sufferers.

They are brain based conditions and, as you know by now, the brain is nothing if not changeable, so some are not necessarily permanent conditions. Other problems such as autism are more of an issue, but many of these kids can develop and survive well given sufficient support and understanding. All have the right to our respect and to achieve happiness.

Condition	Symptoms
Asperger's syndrome	An autism spectrum disorder, people show significant difficulties in social interaction, along with restricted and repetitive patterns of behaviour and interests. Physical clumsiness and atypical use of language are frequently reported.
Attention Deficit & Hyperactivity Disorder ADD or ADHD	Prefrontal cortex is ineffective in separating external and internal states; moving from other directed to self directed; distinguishing the present from the future; delaying gratification. Sufferers are impulsiveness and sometimes hyperactive. They may have poor mental calculation skills, can't wait turns or sit still and limited short term memory.
Auditory Processing Disorder	Deficiency in auditory discrimination and pattern recognition. They may have delayed or mixed up speech for example.
Autism	Autism is a disorder of neural development – information processing in the brain is altered – nerve cells and their synapses connect and organize differently; how this occurs is not well understood.
Brain Tumour	An abnormal growth of cells within the brain, which can be cancerous (malignant) or non-cancerous (benign).
Conduct Disorder	A severe, chronic socially disruptive behaviour pattern. Overlaps with ADD and OPD. Symptoms include inappropriate emotional outbursts and unwillingness to cooperate, consistent verbal abuse, profanity, disruption and intimidation. Sufferers are often moody and hyperactive.

Condition	Symptoms
Depression	A mental condition involving unwanted, intrusive, despair-orientated thoughts.
Dementia	Dementia (meaning "deprived of mind") is a serious loss of cognitive ability in a previously-unimpaired person, beyond what might be expected from normal aging.
Dyslexia	Difficulty with decoding written words, reading comprehension and/or reading fluency.
Anorexia nervosa and bulimia	These are Eating Disorders – Anorexia nervosa is eating too little food through a fear of putting on weight. Bulimia is binge eating then making yourself vomit.
Epilepsy	A common chronic neurological disorder characterized by recurrent seizures.
Multiple Sclerosis	A disease in which the fatty myelin sheaths around the axons of the brain and spinal cord are damaged, leading to demyelination and scarring as well as a broad spectrum of signs and symptoms.
Obsessive Compulsive Disorder	OCD is a psychiatric disorder characterised by anxiety, repetitive thought patterns and rituals.
Oppositional Defiance Disorder	ODD is a psychiatric disorder characterised by abnormal levels of verbal aggressiveness, confrontational attitude and disregard for others' feelings.

Condition	Symptoms
Parkinson's Disease	PD is a degenerative disorder of the CNS that often impairs the sufferer's motor skills, speech, and other functions The primary symptoms are the results of decreased stimulation of the motor cortex by the basal ganglia, usually caused by too little dopamine. PD is both chronic and progressive.
Schizophrenia	A chronic disorder showing a disintegration of the process of thinking and of emotional responsiveness. It often involves 'hearing voices" (auditory hallucinations), paranoid or bizarre delusions, or disorganized speech and thinking.
Stroke	A stroke is caused by a part of the brain being starved of oxygen and the death of some neurons. The effect and the ability to recover depend on the size of the area and its position in the brain.
Tourette Syndrome	TS symptoms include motor and vocal tics. Males are three to four times as likely to have TS as females.

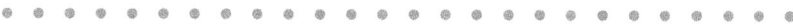

THINK ABOUT IT

* Think about someone you know with a different brain. Will an understanding of how their brain works and its difference to your brain, affect the way you interact with him or her?

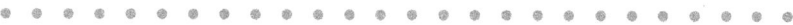

References and Further Reading

BOOKS AND ARTICLES

1. Aamodt, S., Wang S. (2008) *Welcome to Your Brain; the Science of Jet Lag, Love and Other Curiosities of Life*, Rider.

2. Baron-Cohen, S. (2003) *the Essential Difference: The Truth about the Male and Female Brain* Penguin/Basic Books.

3. Biddulph, S. (1998 2nd Ed) *Raising Boys*, Finch.

4. Bradley, M. (2003) *Yes, Your Teen is Crazy*, Harbor Press.

5. Bradley, M. (2004) *Yes, Your Parents are Crazy*, Harbor Press.

6. Carlson, D. (2004) *The Teen Brain Book, Who and What are you?* Bick.

7. Carper, J. (2000) *Your Miracle Brain: Maximize Your Brainpower, Boost Your Memory, Lift Your Mood, Improve Your IQ and Creativity, Prevent and Reverse Mental Aging*, Harper Collins.

8. Carr-Gregg, M, and Shale, E. (2002) *Adolescence*, Finch.

9. Clavier, R. (2009) *Teen Brain Teen Mind: What Parents Need to Know to Survive the Adolescent Years*, Key Porter.

10. Dispenza, J (2007) *Evolve Your Brain, the Science of Changing Your Mind*, Health Communications Inc.

11. Doidge, N. (2007) *The Brain That Changes Itself*, Scribe.

12. Epstein, R. (2010) *Teen 2.0: Saving our Children and Families from the Torment of Adolescence*, Quill Driver.

13. Feinstein, S. (2004) *Secrets of the Teenage Brain*, The Brain Store.

14. Gentile, G. (2010) *Video Games Affect The Brain – For Better*

and Worse. In *Cerebrum: Emerging ideas in Brain Science 2010*. DANA.

15. Giedd, J.N. (2010) *The Teen Brain: Primed to Learn, Primed to Take Risks*, In *Cerebrum: Emerging ideas in Brain Science 2010*. DANA.

16. Gosline, A. (2009) *The 5 Ages of the Brain – and how to get the best out of every stage*, New Scientist No 2702, 4 April 2009.

17. Greenfield, S. (2000) *The Private Life of the Brain*, Penguin.

18. Greenfield, S. (1997) *The Human Brain, a Guided Tour*, Phoenix.

19. Jensen, E. (2000 2nd Ed.) Jenson, Eric (2000) *Brain Based Learning; the New science of Teaching and Training* The Brain Store.

20. Jensen, E. (2000) *Different Brains, Different Learners*, The Brain Store.

21. Jensen, E. (2002) *Introduction to Brain Compatible Education*, Focus Education.

22. Jensen, E., Snider C. (2013) *Turnaround Tools for the Teenage Brain: Helping Underperforming Students Become Lifelong Learners*, Kindle edition, Jossey Bass.

23. Jensen, F.E., Nutt, E (2015) *The Teenage Brain: A neuroscientist's survival guide to raising adolescents and young adults*, Thorsons.

24. Joseph, J. (2008) *Mind your Brain*, Focus Education.

25. Joseph, J. (2002) *Brainy Kids, Brainy Parents*, Focus Education.

26. Katz, L. and Rubin, M. (1999), *Keep Your Brain Alive*, Workman.

27. Medina, J. (2008) *Brain Rules – 12 principles for surviving and thriving at work, home and school*. Pear Press.

28. MacDonald, M. (2008) *Your Brain: the Missing Manual*, Pogue Press.

29. Moore, R. (2015) Inside the Teenage Brain: *How to Parent Strong Willed Children and Adolescents: A Neuroscientist's*

Survival Guide: Raising strong willed child and teenagers, tackling problems with young adults. Kindle edition, RMS Publishing.

30. Morgan, N. (2005) *Blame My Brain: the Amazing Teenage Brain Revealed,* Walker.

31. Ramachandran, VS, (2011) *The Tell-Tale Brain: A Neuroscientist's Quest for what makes us Human,* Norton.

32. Ratey, J. (2001) *A User's Guide to the Brain: Perception, Attention, and the Four Theaters of the Brain,* First Vintage.

33. Restak, R. (2006) *The Naked Brain: How the emerging Neurosociety is Changing how we Live, Work and Love,* Three Rivers Press.

34. Sax, L. (2007) *Boys Adrift: The five factors driving the growing epidemic of unmotivated and underachieving young men.* Basic.

35. Siegel, D.J. (2014) *Brainstorm: The Power and Purpose of the Teenage Brain,* Scribe.

36. Sousa, D. (2001) *How the Brain Learns,* 2nd Ed, Corwin Press.

37. Staunch, B. (2003) *The Primal Teen: What the New Discoveries About the Teenage Brain Tell Us About Our Kids,* Anchor.

38. Walsh, D. (2004) *Why Do They Act That Way? A Survival Guide to the Adolescent Brain for you and Your Teen,* Free Press.

39. Willingham, DT (2009) *Why Don't They Like School?* Jossey-Bass.

40. Willis, J. (2006) *Research Based Strategies to Ignite Student Learning,* ASCD.

41. Willis, J. (2008) *How Your Child Learns Best,* Advantage Quest.

42. Wolfe, P. (2001), *Brain Matters, Translating Research into Classroom Practice,* ASCD.

WEBSITES

1. www.bris.ac.uk/synaptic/basics (excellent animations on how the brain works).

2. www.glycemicindex.com/ Jenny Brand-Miller.

3. www.ncbi.nlm.nih.gov. *Adolescent sleep, school start times, and teen motor vehicle crashes.*

4. www.neurobics.com/exercise.html

5. www.nymag.com, Bonson, Po (2007) *Snooze or Lose* New York Magazine.

6. www.psychiatrictimes.com for information about normal sleep patterns.

7. www.sciencedaily.com *Starting High School One Hour Later May Reduce Teen Traffic Accidents.*

8. www.sleepeducation.net.au, Dr Sarah Blunden.

9. www.sleepfoundation.org/articles.

10. www.sfn.org The Society for Neuroscience.

11. www.epilepsy.org.au/understanding_epilepsy.

12. www.wemmd.com/balance/ Denckla, MB.

13. www.mendosa.com/gilists (for lists of GI values in food).

14. www.webmd.com/fitness-exercise/guide/train-your-brain-with-exercise.

Index

NEED HELP?

Want someone to talk to?

CONTACTS THAT ARE EASY TO REACH:

Counselling services are available for young people who want someone to talk to:

Kids Help Line ph 1800 55 1800
https://kidshelpline.com.au/grownups/contact-us.phpp

Beyond Blue ph 1300 22 4636
https://www.beyondblue.org.au/get-support/get-immediate-support

Or get on line and look up helplines and telephone counselling services in your local area: https://aifs.gov.au/cfca/publications/helplines-and-telephone-counselling-services-children-young-people-and-parents

Bullying and/or cyberbulling

ReachOut: http://au.reachout.com/tough-times/bullying-abuse-and-violence/bullying

Kids Help Line ph 1800 55 1800
https://kidshelpline.com.au/teens/tips/understanding-cyberbullying/

The Author

Derek Pugh is an award-winning author, based in Darwin, in the Northern Territory of Australia. He is an experienced Principal and teacher in both Australian and International Schools, and a Director of Brain Compatible Education International, which teaches students and teachers how brains work and how to use them most efficiently.

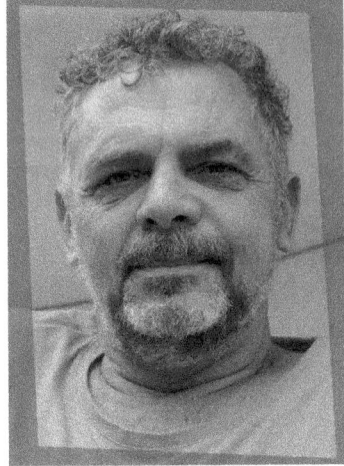

Other Books by Derek Pugh

The British in North Australia 1824-29: Fort Dundas.

Tambora: Travels to Sumbawa and the Mountain that Changed the World.

Tammy Damulkurra.

Turn Left at the Devil Tree.

Carbon Dioxide: Friend or Foe (in publication).

Climate Change and Oceans.
(An ATSE STELR Project (in publication)).

www.ingramcontent.com/pod-product-compliance
Lightning Source LLC
Chambersburg PA
CBHW071436090426
42737CB00011B/1679